Breast cancer

To many women breast cancer is one of the most distressing of all diseases. In a novel departure from other books on the subject, *Breast Cancer* focuses on experiences of the disease from the woman's perspective.

Drawing on 1,000 in-depth interviews, the book makes extensive use of verbatim accounts by women of their own experiences during different stages – from the discovery of the lump, through to diagnosis, treatment, and possible recurrence and death. These extracts – some tragic and poignant, many of them courageous and moving – clearly illustrate the meaning that a diagnosis of breast cancer and its treatment has for different women. A practical, introductory chapter fully describes the medical aspects of the disease. The women's perceptions and insights are interspersed with relevant findings and theories from recent scientific literature.

The authors are well known for their contributions to cancer research and especially for their work on the psychosocial aspects of breast cancer and their effect on the quality of life. Their book is designed to help all those who care for women with breast cancer to understand the distress involved and the means of alleviating some of it. Essential reading for surgeons, radiotherapists and oncologists, *Breast Cancer* will also be immensely helpful to family doctors and nurses, and to students of medicine and health psychology.

The Experience of Illness

Series Editors: Ray Fitzpatrick and Stanton Newman

Breast cancer

Lesley Fallowfield
with
Andrew Clark

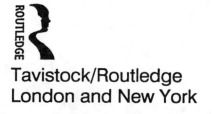

Tavistock/Routledge
London and New York

First published in 1991
by Routledge
11 New Fetter Lane, London EC4P 4EE
29 West 35th Street, New York NY10001

Reprinted 1992

© Chapter 1 1991 Andrew Clark
© Chapters 2–7 1991 Lesley Fallowfield

Typeset by
NWL Editorial Services

Printed and bound in Great Britain by
Biddles Ltd, Guildford and King's Lynn

British Library Cataloguing in Publication Data
Fallowfield, Lesley 1949–
 Breast cancer.
 1. Women. Breasts. Cancer
 I. Title II. Clark, Andrew III. Series
 616.99449

ISBN 0–415–03841–3

For Liz

Contents

Tables

Preface

Over the past six years my research assistants and I have conducted over 1,000 in-depth interviews with women unfortunate enough to be suffering from breast cancer. These women have had to cope with both the knowledge that they have a life-threatening disease and the unpleasant treatments associated with breast cancer. Their responses to these potentially traumatic problems varied enormously. For many women the diagnosis represented a major emotional catastrophe. For others it was yet one more hurdle to overcome, together with many other social iniquities and difficulties apparent in their lives. Certain women viewed the fact of their cancer as a challenge which offered them an opportunity to completely reappraise their attitudes to relationships, work, and life in general. The quotations used throughout this book are all taken from these interviews. Some are tragic and poignant, but many reveal deep personal courage and insight. All illustrate quite clearly the meaning that a diagnosis of breast cancer and its treatment has for different women.

Acknowledgements

I owe an enormous debt to numerous people who have contributed in various ways to either the writing of this book or the research on which it is based. Worthy of special mention is the Cancer Research Campaign which has provided all the financial support for my work on the psychological aspects of breast cancer, for which I thank both the Campaign and all its fund raisers. I am especially indebted to Dr Peter Maguire and Professor Michael Baum who have been my primary research collaborators over the past seven years. Dr Maguire's own research and writing has influenced me greatly. He has probably done more to further the cause of sensible research into the psychological aspects of breast cancer than any other person in this country. It was Dr Maguire who taught me most of what I now know about interviewing people who have cancer. Professor Baum has been a great champion of sound research through clinical trials. He has always been a firm advocate of finding more effective treatments for breast cancer which improve both the quality as well as the quantity of life. Consequently he has done much to promote our work on the psychosocial outcome of therapy amongst his fellow surgeons.

I am also deeply grateful to my indefatigable research assistant and friend, Angela Hall, who has worked so hard over the past four years conducting interviews with patients in our studies. Endless conversations with her about the interpretation of data collected have generated many of the ideas expressed in this book. I also appreciate many of the valuable comments that she made on early drafts.

Little of the research material on which this book is based could have been collected without the encouragement of many surgeons who have helped us gain access to patients. I should particularly like to thank Mr Peter Brooks, Mr Michael Burke, Mr Andrew Clark, Mr Brian Hogbin, Mr Michael Perry and Mr Robert Roxburgh for their valuable co-operation. Needless to say, the examples of bad practice contained in this book are not from interviews with any of their patients! I am also very grateful to breast physician, Dr Anne Rodway, for her active help and encouragement with the work on mammographic screening.

My secretary, Ruth Sutton, deserves a special mention and thanks for her diligent help with all aspects of my work, but particularly for the uncomplaining manner in which she always seems to manage to transcribe my scribbles and jottings miraculously into a well-prepared manuscript.

I should also like to thank the two editors of the series, Dr Stan Newman and Dr Ray Fitzpatrick, first, for asking me to contribute and second, for their constructive criticisms and helpful suggestions during the preparation of the book.

Finally, the unsung heroines of this book are, of course, the hundreds of courageous women who have given up their time to talk about their experiences of breast cancer. I thank them all and hope that their insightful comments have been conveyed accurately by me and, more importantly, in a manner likely to help all those who care for women with breast cancer to understand more about the distress involved and the means of alleviating some of it.

Lesley Fallowfield 1990

Editors' preface

Breast cancer is the most common form of cancer for women. As screening becomes more established, both survival and quality of life for this disease may be dramatically improved. The experiences and decisions of women in relation to attendance for screening and early identification of symptoms are one central issue developed in this book. The discovery of a diagnosis of breast cancer creates enormous distress for the woman and for her family. For women with breast cancer there are potentially complex decisions to be faced about treatment options. These decisions are not helped by the changing policies for radical versus conservative interventions and the lack of firm evidence to direct choice.

Lesley Fallowfield is uniquely placed to write this book. Over a number of years she has carried out some of the most important and innovative research in this area. In order to assess the impact of breast cancer, she has used methods of research which depend on acute sensitivity to women's own accounts and understandings. She also brings to bear another area of expertise and research experience – the critical issue of quality of life in health care. Andrew Clark provides an up-to-date explanation of medical and surgical aspects of breast cancer.

This book is a rich analysis of the experience of breast cancer. One central theme is the woman's perspective when receiving the diagnosis, and subsequently as information about implications is assimilated, and the meaning of the diagnosis is negotiated with others. Lesley Fallowfield has introduced, and discusses here, novel techniques to enhance patients' understanding of their diagnosis and its implications. The authors critically examine conventional understanding of the relative importance of threats posed by cancer compared with the fears of disfigurement that might arise from surgery. We are reminded by the authors of the concerns women face regarding the threat of return of the disease and of the difficulties of coping with recurrence. This is not a pessimistic analysis and is a powerful statement for health professionals of the scope for positive interventions.

What is breast cancer and how is it treated? A surgeon's experience of breast cancer

Epidemiology and causation

Cancer of the breast occurs in women of all races and appears to have happened throughout history. It is slowly increasing in frequency all over the western world. In Britain about 24,000 new cases are diagnosed each year, and 15,000 deaths are certified as due to the disease. This suggests that about a third of all cases die of some other cause, with no evidence of further cancer in their bodies. These women could reasonably be claimed to have been cured of their breast cancer. To put it another way, 1 woman in 14 will contract breast cancer during her lifetime and 1 in 21 will die of it (Cancer Research Campaign 1988).

Britain tops the international table, alas, with a death rate five times that of Japan. Now that there is a lot of information on migrant populations, we know that Japanese who emigrate to America soon share American death rates for most common cancers. While this has not yet come true for breast cancer, there is evidence to suggest that it will. Thus the information from migration suggests that environmental factors play a large part in the onset of the disease. Despite intensive study, it is disappointing to report that no clear guidance as to how to reduce risk through diet has emerged.

Those factors implicated in the development of breast cancer that can be avoided are obesity and ionizing radiation. Of the remaining risk factors, age is inevitable and some others carry such a small risk that few would wish to change their lives because of them. It may be more important to list some common worries which are presently under investigation and have not been shown to affect significantly the incidence of the disease. They include high fat diet, hormone replacement therapy, oral contraception, alcohol, stress, and benign breast disease.

Even where an association between a causative factor and raised breast cancer incidence is shown, it would be simplistic to assume that a commonsense response, such as dietary change, is likely to produce a benefit. Much of the cause is built into our systems over a timescale of 20–40 years.

Heredity has a large part to play in some cases. One or two close relatives with the disease increase a woman's risk three or four times. If the cluster is close enough, the effect is greater, so that a woman with mother and sister affected is very likely indeed to develop breast cancer, and at a younger than average age (Stoll 1989).

Pathology and staging

Breast cancer is a term which covers a very wide variety of disease patterns. At the extremes, some patients' cancers remain confined to the breast for years, while others have no lump to feel in the breast, becoming ill with severe metastatic disease elsewhere in the body. Nevertheless the majority of patients follow the broad middle path described below.

The cells lining the breast ducts and forming the secretory groups are normally orderly both in content and arrangement. Incipient cancer is recognizable by characteristic calcification on X-ray of the breast, or by microscopic examination of tissue taken for diagnosis, or as part of an operation to remove a true cancer. The condition is fully curable by surgery but may affect both breasts. This situation is comparable to the finding of abnormal cells on the surface of the cervix, curable by excision or vaporization of the tissue. Since it has no outward manifestation, this phase of breast cancer has only been noticed incidentally in the past, but its ability to produce X-ray signs means it is being found more frequently now. This produces new dilemmas for doctors and patients. It is not known how many breast cancers may start in this way or how long this phase of the disease may last.

The cells of an active cancer are demonstrably malignant by their ability to travel to unusual sites. Thus they grow outward into the breast tissue, entering the blood and lymphatic vessels where loose cells travel with the stream of fluid to distant sites.

Local growth, or invasion, excites support tissues, namely the blood vessels and fibre cells, to grow in unison. Thus a lump appears in the softer surrounding tissue. On an X-ray the radiating strands of growth are characteristic, as are the sharp spicules of calcium which often accompany them. Over 70 per cent of all cancers can be seen on X-ray before they can be felt and this is the basis of mammography. If neglected, invasive cancers grow up into the skin, starving the circulation, and produce ulceration. Eventually, redness, thickening, and tumour deposits occur over a wide area of chest wall, while invasion of the armpit produces lymphatic obstruction with painful swelling of the arm.

Metastasis is the appearance of a mass of cancer in another part of the body at a distance from the original cancer. Thus the original lump is the primary and all the metastases are secondaries. Loose cells in the lymph vessels of the breast are trapped in the armpit (axillary) lymph nodes and form secondaries there. As these secondaries enlarge, they either release cells themselves or cause cells from the primary to by-pass them in new lymphatic channels. Hence nodes further from the tumour become involved, such as those in the root of the neck.

Malignant cells may also find their way to the glands behind the breastbone – the internal mammary nodes. In either case node metastases may release cells into the blood stream. Similarly many breast cancers invade blood vessels directly. The great majority of loose cells in the circulation die off, but some lodge in distant tissues and start to grow into tumour masses. The most likely sites for breast metastases are: bone, lung, liver, brain, the ovary, and adrenal. Each gives a different group of symptoms.

Bone secondaries replace the bone marrow, giving rise to anaemia in a few patients. In the majority they produce symptoms by weakening the bone, with pain, spinal deformity, or sudden fracture of major bones. Occasionally the tumour mass or deformity of the spine leads to compression of the spinal cord, with paralysis. This can be relieved by removal of the posterior plate – a procedure known as a laminectomy.

Lung secondaries produce few symptoms when confined to the lung tissue, but they often invade the pleura coating the lung, which renders it inelastic. At the same time quantities of fluid appear, further compressing the lung, and causing increased breathlessness.

Liver secondaries cause uncomfortable enlargement, press on the veins causing fluid to accumulate in the abdomen, and eventually replace enough liver tissue to prevent normal liver function. At this stage jaundice may appear.

Brain secondaries produce neurological impairment appropriate to their site and also a general rise in intracerebral pressure. Ovarian metastases are symptomless, but those in the adrenal, like some of our treatments, can produce shortages of the normal hormones. The apathy and vomiting can be reversed by steroid administration, with considerable symptom relief.

Cancer cells are greedy cuckoos, consuming an unfair share of the circulating nutrients in the bloodstream. By the time the original one cell has grown to produce two kilograms of tumour, much of the rest of the patient's tissue has wasted away, three years have passed, and the body and spirit can continue no more. The exact mode of death in cancer patients who have avoided specific problems is hard to understand.

Staging

In order to facilitate comparisons and simplify care, all professionals now use the International Classification which may be summarized as follows:

T1 tumours are 2 cm or less.
T2 tumours are between 2–5 cm.
T3 tumours are over 5 cm.
T4 tumours are fixed to the chest wall or skin and are of any size.

The classification further considers the armpit glands which can often be felt in their normal state, so:

N1 are mobile axillary nodes.
N2 are fixed axillary nodes.
N3 are nodes in the neck, or a swollen arm.

Finally, if there are no signs of metastases elsewhere in the body, we write M0, and if there are, M1.

All these assessments are subjective, depending on who looks, how hard they look, and what with.

Diagnosis and investigation

Since four out of five patients with breast lumps seen in surgical clinics do not have cancer it is important to categorize them accurately and quickly, with the greatest sensitivity.

Some breast cancers can be diagnosed almost entirely by clinical examination; dimpling of the skin, thickened skin, and swollen glands in the armpit or neck show that the lump is malignant.

The mainstay of investigation is needle aspiration cytology. In some districts it may be necessary to perform a biopsy, that is remove a piece of the lump either by operation or with a special thick-cutting needle. Either test is backed up by a mammogram: an X-ray of both breasts to characterize the known lump and discover any other suspicious areas.

Most women with breast lumps realize their potential significance and are very frightened. The rest of this book will have much to say about the experiences of those with cancer. Those women who do not have cancer suffer the same anguish until they can be fully reassured. We all know that it is more difficult to prove a negative than a positive. Thus women with benign lumps may have a negative needle test, with 1 chance in 20 of having cancer nevertheless. Then they may undergo mammography with cheering news thereafter, but still 1 chance in 5 or 10 that the diagnosis has been missed. Hence the cloud is lifting through one or two outpatient visits, but it is often only fully dispelled when the lump is surgically removed and the final report from the microscopist is read out to them. Any who doubt the stress related to having a benign lump should watch a woman's face as she hears the report, and her stride as she leaves the clinic.

Planning treatment

By now the women with cancer will have been told their diagnosis and had a week or so to recover from the news and consider the treatment options. The patients' thoughts during this stressful period form the substance of Chapter 3; so what are the surgeons thinking?

First, they know that smallish lumps are unlikely to have spread elsewhere in the body, but the patient is nevertheless asked to undergo chest X-ray and blood tests if these have not already been done. Meanwhile, surgeon and patient can discuss the treatment options.

Most surgeons know that the choice of initial treatment for the affected breast does not influence outcome in terms of survival. They also know that many women hope to keep their breast and be treated by lumpectomy and radiotherapy. Unfortunately, 30 to 50 per cent of lumps are unsuitable for this treatment by virtue of their size or proximity to the nipple. The surgeons know that putting more people in this treatment group can lead to future trouble. As it is, about 15 per cent of patients having lumpectomy with radiotherapy will have further cancer at the site of the first lump, and undergo mastectomy up to three years later (Locker *et al.* 1989). Performing more lumpectomies in the fringe group seems certain to increase the risk of local recurrence. The lumpectomy patients in the large American trial had fewer late mastectomies, probably because the microscopist were not happy with the initial excision in some cases, and the surgeon did an immediate mastectomy at the time of the lumpectomy in 10 per cent of cases (Fisher *et al.* 1985).

Surgeons who are happy to discuss the options with their patients also know that about 30 per cent of those suitable for either operation will choose a mastectomy (Fallowfield *et al.* 1990). The number will vary depending on the way in which the information in the previous paragraph is presented to the patient. Mastectomy, of course, gives a chance of avoiding radiotherapy, which patients find as debilitating as surgery.

Whichever operation is eventually chosen, it is increasingly important to remove some of the axillary lymph nodes as the presence of cancer in the nodes is an important pointer to the higher probability of future metastasis. When there is more risk extra treatment will be indicated.

Why operate at all? Most of those who care for breast cancer patients live in dread of uncontrolled disease on the chest wall and know that well-planned treatment can minimize this. Many women, particularly in France, have been treated by radiotherapy alone, but British radiotherapists prefer the lump to be removed first, not only because it improves the results of treatment but also because of the added information from the microscopy of the lump and glands. Some elderly patients can be managed successfully by therapy with hormone tablets, such as Tamoxifen, alone. The lump often ceases to grow, and sometimes disappears. Unfortunately, some lumps do not shrink, or they start to grow again later, so the treatment is less suitable for patients with serious hopes of cure. The tablets also provide a useful psychological stopgap between diagnosis and treatment in many younger patients.

'Never define your terms,' said Professor Popper, 'you will spoil a good argument.' So it goes with the value of different treatments for breast cancer and axillary glands. Broadly speaking, we have moved from an era of supersurgery – the radical and supraradical mastectomies – to more conservative surgery which calls for more radiotherapy and a willingness to accept local recurrence as the price of cosmetic acceptability. The biological consequences of increased rates of local recurrence are probably insignificant – just as many patients are alive and well five to ten years after initial diagnosis by one method of treatment as another. Patients are understandably very distressed by local recurrence. While surgeons and radiotherapists find it very disappointing, they can usually offer further useful, and possibly curative, treatment.

Management by lumpectomy requires close co-operation, so a pre-operative visit to the radiotherapist for assessment is very helpful, as are counselling sessions with a trained counsellor/breast nurse. Patients with larger breast lumps (over 5 cm diameter) are known to be incurable and are managed in the same way as those with metastases.

Through all these considerations, somehow our patient, surgeon, counsellor, and radiotherapist have agreed an initial treatment. Unlike the organs deeper in the body, the diagnosis cannot be withheld, nor the consequences of treatment lightly dismissed. The surgeon is beginning a new long-term relationship with the patient, in the worst of circumstances. Success is measured not in increased survival, but in the founding of trust through honesty and compassion. Stress for the surgeon comes through the repeated process of diagnosis and discussion, watching the hope fade from the patient's eyes. A general surgeon working in a district general hospital may go through this process between two and six times a week, year after year. It is no wonder that many avoid the challenge of open discussion by retiring into a professional shell of starch, euphemism, and 'being busy'. Strangely, there is no structured psychological support for them, their training and background being at the 'organic' end of the spectrum of care.

Diagnosis and operations

To those who deal regularly in the technical side of care, there is no mystery. Past patients, however, hide their scars thoroughly, so new patients do not know what to expect. For some, there are great fears. It is important for the professionals to remember this and give clear simple explanations of each procedure.

Diagnostic procedures

Aspiration cytology can be done simply in outpatients, without any anaesthetic. The needle used is the same as that used for drawing a blood sample.

Needle biopsy requires some local anaesthetic and a 3–4 mm incision in the skin. Through this is passed a needle about 3 mm across, with an internal sliding section. This allows solid cores of suspicious areas to be withdrawn. The process is easier if the needle action is mechanized either manually or with a spring-loaded handle.

Surgery

Open biopsy is definitely an operation – usually under general anaesthetic, in an operating theatre. Usually an excision biopsy is done, meaning that the whole lump is removed for analysis. Sometimes cancers found in this way require no further surgery, only radiotherapy. When the suspicious area is only visible on X-ray, and cannot be felt, the procedure is called 'localization' and is more complicated. First, the radiologist inserts a thin wire marker in the breast tissue, and repeats the X-rays. She or he then gives guidance to the surgeon as to where the suspicious area lies in relation to the marker. The area is then excised under general anaesthetic. The excised part is re-X-rayed for confirmation before the operation is concluded.

Wide excision, sometimes called tylectomy, implies the planned excision of the lump together with an area of surrounding breast tissue. This is the standard operation for patients being treated conservatively. Many phrases are used to describe this operation: wide local excision and tylectomy both imply removal of an area of normal-looking tissue around the malignant mass, while local excision, lumpectomy, and breast conservation do not distinguish the closeness of the excision margin. Segmental mastectomy is either a synonym for wide excision, or implies powers of surgical dissection unknown to ordinary surgeons.

Simple mastectomy, sometimes called total mastectomy, is probably the commonest operation for breast cancer. It involves removal of an area of skin, including the nipple, and all the breast tissue. The lower lymph glands in the axilla are also removed to aid management decisions. After the operation there is a simple scar leaving a flat chest wall.

Radical mastectomy implies the planned removal of all the breast, nipple, and one or two muscles joining the ribs to the shoulder bones. This allows wide access to the axilla with the intention of removing all its glands in a single mass along with the breast. This has a similar value to radiotherapy in that area. Because of the muscle loss the deformity is greater, and there is a risk of chronic arm swelling. It may be helpful to remember that radical mastectomy was invented before radiotherapy, to treat lumps considerably larger than those commonly seen today. Subsequently, simple mastectomy with radiotherapy became the standard treatment, slowly losing the radiotherapy element in favourable cases. Radiotherapy improved and came back into its own with a reduction in surgery from mastectomy to lumpectomy. The future surely holds lumpectomy without radiotherapy.

Cutting into a woman's breast is not as easy as many more complex operations. The soft mobile tissues constantly challenge the spatial assumptions of the surgeon. Firmer but benign tissue draws surgeons into removal of unnecessarily larger areas. The main technical complication is bleeding into the wound. It can be reduced by multiple stitches in the deeper tissues, or by drainage of a wound for a day or so. Drains tend to increase hospital stay, creating a dilemma for all. Happily, plastic or absorbable skin sutures improve scar appearance and make stitch removal easy or unnecessary.

Patients stay a day or less for biopsy, a few days for wide excision, and a week or more for mastectomy. Mastectomy patients meet the breast nurse specialist again in the ward, and can discuss their feelings with her, and be given a light, temporary prosthetic breast before departure. Many lumpectomy patients may not yet be fully informed, since microscopists' reports generally take four to eight days and they will have left the hospital by then. Nevertheless, they will be as distressed, or more so, as those who know their diagnoses and all are in great need of counselling at this stage.

Breast reconstruction

In those women for whom breast loss creates psychological distress breast reconstruction is available. The breast tissue can be substituted by a plastic sac. It is often appropriate to start with an empty sac which can be progressively filled with fluid through an injection port under the nearby skin. Once the correct size is reached, a small operation removes the first sac and substitutes a permanent and more natural one. Problems include migration of the sac to the wrong place, hardening of the scar round the sac, lack of nipple, and difficulty in diagnosing local recurrence of the breast cancer. The ingenuity of plastic surgeons has produced an array of choices in re-forming the lost breast tissue and skin. Detailed descriptions are not appropriate here, but the principles are easy to describe.

New skin and tissue can be found on the back or abdomen and, keeping the blood vessels intact, swung around to form a new breast mound. Problems include scarring at the original site, failure of the blood supply, and lack of nipple.

Either of these reconstructive procedures can be performed early, or after a couple of years. The happiness brought about by improved body shape may be spoilt by dissatisfaction with the appearance, anxiety about recurrence, and failure of the change to produce the desired social effect. By and large, surgeons are increasingly willing to reconstruct early in suitable cases.

Adjuvant radiotherapy, hormones, chemotherapy

After the initial cancer operation, the microscopist's report is reviewed and decisions on future care made according to the unit's policy. Most lumpectomy patients and some mastectomy patients will be recommended to have radiotherapy, normally on an outpatient basis. Sessions are painless, happening every weekday for three to six weeks. Extra treatment is given to the lumpectomy area itself, either by more external beam therapy, or occasionally with implants. Under anaesthetic the surgeon or radiotherapist places plastic tubes in the breast tissue, and subsequently radioactive material is placed in the tubes for a suitable time, usually a few hours. Afterwards the tubes are withdrawn and the remainder of the treatment given by external beam, using gamma-rays from a cobalt source, or X-rays from a generator. These are effectively the same.

Nobody knows exactly who needs radiotherapy. Without it, local recurrence happens sooner and more frequently. It could, of course, be reserved for when that happens, especially as no area of the body can undergo a second course of treatment. Although it seems instinctively good to avoid as many local recurrences as possible, it is clearly bad to give unnecessary and debilitating treatment. Our knowledge as to which patients to treat is poor, but we do know that overall survival is unaffected by radiation given early to all, rather than later to those who need it. Radiotherapists prefer to treat tissue with a few cancer cells in it than with lumps, so early treatment for high risk areas seems wise (Berstock *et al.* 1985). The side effects of radiotherapy include red, sore skin, tiredness, and nausea. Later the arm may swell and the skin of the irradiated area becomes thin, shiny, and hairless. Occasionally there are symptoms of radiation change in deeper organs – rib necrosis, lung fibrosis, and a small increase in the chance of heart disease.

The techniques and equipment are fast improving, so that the experience and results are far better than they once were.

All treatment of the 'just in case' character is called adjuvant, though occasionally the word prophylactic appears. This concept continues with hormone manipulations. The specialized cells of the sex organs and breasts are particularly dependent on the circulating sex hormones which are produced by the adrenals and gonads (ovaries or testes). Identical treatment concepts to those outlined below therefore apply to men with cancer of the prostate. Years ago surgeons knew that removing the ovaries of pre-menopausal women could produce remission in active breast cancer. Trials of ovarian removal at the time of initial treatment suggested a long-term benefit. Nowadays ovarian function can be stopped by a small dose of radiotherapy. Consequent upon the clinical observation, a drug called Tamoxifen or Nolvadex was synthesized by ICI. This blocks the uptake of oestrogen by the breast tissue, be it normal or cancerous. In laboratory tests it also seemed to have an anti-cancer effect in the absence of oestrogen. In clinical practice it has been helpful in the treatment of the elderly, as I mentioned, but also as adjuvant therapy in the majority of breast cancer patients. It not only defers the onset of recurrence anywhere in the body, but confers a benefit in survival which continues from our initial experience to the present day – about ten years.

Sex hormones are also produced by the adrenal gland. Their output can be blocked by a drug called Aminoglutethimide. This appears more difficult to manage, and is still under study.

The third arm of adjuvant treatment is the use of anticancer drugs – chemotherapy. For some time after the initial value of this form of treatment was shown, there was concern that the action occurred indirectly. It was possible that ovarian and adrenal function was arrested by the drugs rather than their having a direct effect on the tumour themselves. This has now been sorted out, and women at high risk of recurrence, before the menopause, get long-term advantages from treatment with a triple cocktail of Cyclophosphamide, Methotrexate, and 5–Fluorouracil. Repeated courses are given over a six-month period. This treatment often has unpleasant side-effects such as hair loss, nausea and vomiting, and loss of resistance to infections.

Again we are faced with the problem of who needs which treatment (National Institutes of Health 1985). One solution has been to test the cancer cells for the presence and quantity of oestrogen receptors on their cell surface. The patient could then be classified into high and low to discover if hormone therapy has been more beneficial in the high receptor group or not. Results have been conflicting, so that in some centres the test is used as a guide to treatment, in others not. Another more traditional approach is for the microscopist to assess the virulence of the tumour by counting the number of actively dividing cells.

Whatever the choice of adjuvant therapy it eventually ceases – and we all wait.

Follow-up and recurrence

Regular attendance and examination are required of, or requested by, most cancer patients. The interviews and examinations are conducted by surgeons or radiotherapists at intervals ranging from twelve weeks at first to a year later. The traditional visit and examination have been shown to be oddly ineffective, as only one in three recurrences are found by examination or enquiry at that time. Patients often find their own recurrences, perhaps through knowing where to look. In addition, much of the depression and anxiety catalogued later in this book is not recognized by surgeons or seen as their problem. Many surgeons are unaware of the symptoms of depression, while some feel it is an inevitable consequence of the diagnosis and treatment, and is beyond help. This difficulty extends also to general practitioners.

The visit seems to provide reassurance for both patient and doctor, but this may only be as a consequence of the anxiety generated in the lead-up to it. Perhaps the most significant part of follow-up is regular mammography of the other breast to discover any small new cancer there. In future it may be possible to do this through the general breast screening programme.

For some patients, then, confidence in survival grows as the shock of mutilation and threat of death recede. Visits are less frequent, more of a reunion and a secret celebration of success. Others demonstrate their anxiety by repeated attendances to discuss various bodily symptoms which need reassurance and sometimes investigation. Such is the plethora of possible patterns of recurrence that this area is a minefield for the unwary doctor who must find a path between unnecessary repetition of investigations and blasé reassurance.

Investigations are not routinely performed on all patients. The interval between an altered investigation and the appearance of symptoms is 6–8 weeks, so an advocate of regularly repeated investigations would be hard put to suggest a realistic interval between retests. If the patient is not suffering symptoms from a secondary then there seems little value in advancing the moment of diagnosis, with loss of expectation of a happy life. All treatment methods eventually fail, often in proportion to the length of time they have been applied. Starting early to treat a symptomless secondary could only be of value in a few circumstances, for instance threat of spinal or long bone fracture. These are rare in the symptomless patient and do not therefore give a useful general policy. A proportion of chest wall recurrences found clinically may be treated and returned to the potentially cured group. The remainder of these and all those patients with proof of widespread recurrent cancer are condemned to die. Routine investigation of symptomless patients is therefore pointless.

The race to prove recurrence is appropriate if a patient is symptomatic and concerned. Her mental problems are as strong or stronger than those of a worried person with an initial breast lump. Her understanding of the disease is greater so she probably knows that her next serious symptom is of great significance.

All treatments are now palliative. The art of the oncologist/radio-therapist and surgeon lies in devising appropriate plans to reduce symptoms and prolong useful life. The useful treatment methods have already been described and examples of a few common strategies will be given.

Surgery has considerable value in controlling chest wall recurrence, especially in previously irradiated areas. Orthopaedic surgeons and neurosurgeons relieve crumbling spines, and the miseries of threatened or actual long bone fracture can be alleviated by metal reinforcement.

Radiotherapy toughens soft bone secondaries instead of, or after, orthopaedic repair. In younger women it is undoubtedly the kindest way to reduce ovarian function. It has great value in treating further tumour areas causing specific problems, especially those apparent to the patient. It is not good, we suspect, to feel or see your lump growing. Hormone therapy may already have been applied as Tamoxifen, up to the time of recurrence. Alternatives include high-dose progesterone treatment with Megestrol, or further reduction of the patient's own hormone output with Aminoglutethimide. Surgeons have, in the past, pursued the endocrine glands with great determination and ingenuity. Thus women with recurrent disease were subjected to bilateral adrenalectomy or removal of the pituitary. Either operation led to disquieting imbalances of other hormones requiring a vast array of tablets and antidiuretic hormone injections to keep the body organized. The surgical enthusiasm seemed to be at times an alternative to a realistic and sympathetic discussion with all concerned. Certainly, it was hard to see how filling the patient's last few months with major surgery could enhance her quality of life. The odd success did not seem to justify the many failures.

Very similar considerations apply to the use of chemo-therapy. What is success? Which of us could come between a determined patient desperate for relief, and the consequences of her choice?

Acknowledgement of therapeutic failure is often received with relief by baffled patients. Realistic discussions with the patient and relatives, attended by as many members of the caring team as possible, can pave the way for a kind and effective terminal care plan. Nowadays few hospital or family doctors can match the skill of a professional symptom control and terminal care specialist.

Hospice and domiciliary specialist nursing care and counselling produces a social and therapeutic plan far in advance of the ad hoc arrangements of twenty-five years ago. I would not belittle the successes of family doctors who take a full and proper interest in the process of dying, and give their patients a wonderful service. They are, alas, in the minority.

Talking about trials

Most biological observations are more subjective than we think. Send ten trusty surgeons to describe the same breast lump, and the answers are so different as to suggest ten lumps and one surgeon rather than the reverse. Thousands of publications on the subject of breast cancer fail to contribute useful knowledge because they ignore this and similar findings – all grouped under the heading of 'Observer error'. If we hope to test a new treatment we can only make progress by the intellectual rigour of the controlled trial. Observer errors are distributed by a random process to each arm of the trial. One arm must be the best current treatment (which was of course the 'winner' of the previous trial) and the new treatment forms the other.

After five years we will have a good idea about the value of the new treatment in terms of recurrence rates and after ten years death rates. Meanwhile other trials will be started, finished and published, and so on.

In Britain only 8 per cent of patients enter trials of primary treatment, probably through a lack of enthusiasm among surgeons. Perhaps the commonest reason offered by these surgeons is a desire to offer clear and unambiguous advice to their frightened and unhappy patients. More recently, and for good reasons, society has gone as far as requiring all trials to be explained fully to patients before entry. This has proved too much for many breast surgeons and patients, with consequent reduction in the rate at which new knowledge can be tested and applied. We are left with another salutary reminder. Many patients who appear to have been given information about a trial before entry did not feel they had a choice. I have a growing feeling that the sophistication and wisdom of these brave women with breast cancer may yet surprise the ethicists who have brought forward this new problem. The paradox is that specialist cancer centres enter more patients in trials, and yet attract more patients.

Conclusion

Earlier presentation with smaller lumps, screening programmes, and improvements in technology for diagnosis and treatment are important changes. Smaller operations likewise help, but a further important advance we could offer is more sympathetic care for our brave and unhappy patients. Fearful of losing their social contacts, under-diagnosed psychologically and never 'twenty-one again', it is no wonder that our patients either idolize their surgeons or fall into deep despair. Neither should be necessary.

Chapter two

Lay attitudes, beliefs, screening, and self-examination

The number of instances in which malignant disease of the breast and uterus follows immediately antecedent emotion of a depressing character is too large to be set down to chance, or to the general liability to the buffets of ill-fortune which the cancer patients, in the passage through life, share with most other people not so afflicted.

(Snow 1893)

The introductory chapter showed that both the etiology and biology of breast cancer is still rather poorly understood. This can make it difficult at times to challenge some of the popular myths and fears that lay people often harbour about causal factors, prevalence of the disease, and its curability relative to other life-threatening illnesses. However, an appreciation of some of these lay attitudes and beliefs about breast cancer has important implications for the utilization of screening services and the psychological aspects of patient care. In this chapter, therefore, I shall describe some of the commonly-held fears about cancer and look at the most frequently cited beliefs about causal factors.

Fears and beliefs about cancer

Knowledge about prevalence

Cancer is regarded with more or less universal dread; several population surveys have shown that it is perceived with more alarm and considered more serious than any other disease. Even though heart disease is responsible for more deaths, almost 60 per cent of women sampled in 1966 thought that cancer killed more people than any other disease (Briggs and Wakefield 1966).

Despite this pessimistic view of the likely mortality figures, over two-thirds of the sample questioned thought cancer curable to a certain extent, although only 44 per cent had ever heard of anyone being cured of their disease.

In a later study, almost three-quarters of those questioned thought cancer curable, and more than half knew of an individual who had survived cancer (Knopf 1974). Both of these studies were conducted on women living in the UK, but data from the American Cancer Society survey in 1973, which explored beliefs about breast cancer in over 1,000 women, revealed similar misconceptions, including an exaggerated estimate of the prevalence of the disease, with over half the sample thinking that it affected at least one in ten women. Over a third (38 per cent) questioned thought that breast lumps were more likely to be malignant than benign.

All the studies mentioned above were conducted over fifteen years ago. Breast cancer now has a much higher profile in terms of the numbers of articles that have appeared in newspapers and magazines together with the many television and radio programmes. Consequently, one might suppose that knowledge about the disease amongst lay populations has improved. In a recent research project involving 122 asymptomatic women attending a breast cancer screening clinic in South London, myths and misconceptions about the disease were still very apparent (Fallowfield et al. 1990). Despite the fact that people tend to overestimate the incidence of cancer in general, the women in this study severely underestimated the risks of a woman getting breast cancer, with only 14 per cent knowing that breast cancer affects about one in every twelve women. Over one-third of the women did not know that most breast lumps are not due to cancer and 5 per cent thought that cancer was the cause of the majority of breast lumps. The women attending the breast screening clinic had been sent an information leaflet, together with their letter of invitation, so it was also disappointing to discover that the majority failed to appreciate that the chance of a breast lump being cancer increases as a woman gets older. Latest available statistics (HMSO 1986) show that incidence rates rise from less than 10 per 100,000 in women aged 30 years or under to 300 per 100,000 in women aged over 85 years. Only 1 per cent of our sample thought that risks increase for women over the age of 65 years.

Causal factors

Table 2.1 provides a summary of some of the causal factors considered most relevant by lay people in the development of breast cancer. It should be noted that both symptomatic and asymptomatic women hold similar beliefs. On both sides of the Atlantic the most frequently cited causal factor was a knock or injury. Significant numbers of women also attribute breast cancer to smoking, heredity, infection, or life-style, including immorality. More recently, doubtless spurred on by media hype, many women cite 'stress' as the primary factor. Noxious life events are an explanation frequently found in the literature, as can be seen at the beginning of this chapter, in the quotation written by Snow almost a century ago. Anecdotal evidence that stress provoked by life's traumas is responsible for breast cancer is readily available, but demonstrating this in a scientifically acceptable manner is fraught with many methodological difficulties which will be discussed later.

In our study a questionnaire assessing knowledge about causal factors in the development of breast cancer produced some interesting findings (Fallowfield *et al.* 1990). Many women knew that heredity may play some part in the development of breast cancer, with 49 per cent of the sample realizing that having relatives with breast cancer tends to increase one's own risk. However, the small but significant increase in risk due to nulliparity was mentioned by only 6 per cent. The wide publicity in the spring of 1989, following the publication of a report in the *Lancet* showing a link with the contraceptive pill, clearly had an impact on the women questioned, as 40 per cent felt that taking the pill placed one at risk from breast cancer (Chilvers *et al.* 1989). Increasing age was not recognized as a major risk factor, as was evident by the fact that merely 25 per cent of the sample felt that having passed the menopause placed one at risk. A surprisingly high number (35 per cent) of the sample thought

Table 2.1 Lay beliefs of causal factors in breast cancer

Knocks, bumps, or strains
Infection
Heredity
Stress
Divine retribution or punishment
Life-style
Smoking
Taking contraceptive pills

that being hit in the breast was an important causal factor in the disease.

These data were collected from asymptomatic women attending for mammographic screening, but what of women who have a confirmed diagnosis of breast cancer? Fallowfield *et al.* interviewed 269 women with breast cancer in a prospective study with a three-year follow-up (1990). The selection of quotations below is taken from interviews with women in this study. They illustrate the point that the primary factors considered important by a lay population of women in the development of cancer are remarkably similar whether or not symptoms are present.

Knocks, bumps, and strains

Many asymptomatic women thought that being hit in the breast was a causal factor. Likewise, several women with a diagnosis of cancer in our study claimed that various knocks, bumps, and strains had caused their breast lumps

> I just found this lump when I was washing, then I remembered bumping my breast on a door handle three months ago. I told the doctor that's what caused it, but he didn't agree with me.

> I'd been carrying a heavy bag all day which must have pulled a muscle or something. It was still sore three months later when I went to the doctor.

> I noticed a slight swelling after I had lifted a drum of glue at the school that I work at.

> I'd had this lump for a while, but I'd hurt my back when I was decorating, so I thought that it was something to do with that.

> It was the seat belt in a car accident that caused it.

One reason why so many women cite trauma as a cause of cancer could be due to the fact that a knock or strain makes them rub the breast, and in so doing they find a lump which has probably been present for some time. The women then wrongly interpret the cancer as the consequence of the antecedent traumatic event.

Infection

Some women may attribute the development of cancer to previous infection such as mastitis.

I've suffered from mastitis all my life, so I'm not surprised I've got cancer now.

The notion that cancer itself is contagious and that one can catch it from another sufferer is occasionally mentioned.

I'd been working as a cleaner at an old people's home and lots of them died of cancer. I suppose I could have picked something up there, couldn't I?

Fears about the possibility that cancer is contagious was examined in a lay population by Verres (1986). Although few people explicitly stated that they thought cancer contagious, Verres found that precise questioning about the degrees of intimacy that people were prepared to engage in with the victims of cancer produced some surprising responses. Many stated that they would refuse to eat anything cooked by someone with cancer. Over a third of the people interviewed would not share a drinking utensil with anyone suffering from cancer and many more admitted that they would avoid direct physical contact with such patients. Women with breast cancer frequently express the fear that they will be left to die a painful, lonely death and there is evidence that their worries are not merely paranoia. Peters-Golden's study in 1982 of women with breast cancer showed that 50 per cent of the women felt that people now avoided them. She also found that 61 out of 100 healthy women said they would avoid contact with a friend with cancer. It is of course entirely possible that many people avoid seeing relatives and friends with cancer because they find the experience too distressing to confront. However, it is important for all those working in the field of oncology to understand that the profound ignorance surrounding the possible modes of transmission may well contribute to a patient's social isolation from family and friends. Thus, health carers and health educationists should work harder to allay the myths and fears that cancer is necessarily contagious.

Heredity

The risk of developing breast cancer increases two- to three-fold if first degree relatives, i.e., mother, aunts, or sisters of a woman have the disease. This risk increases fourteen-fold if both the mother and sister of a woman have breast cancer (Sattin *et al.* 1985). Some of the women interviewed in our study felt that having other relatives with cancer of any site was a significant factor in the development of breast cancer.

> My mother was 45 and she got these headaches – it was a brain tumour that killed her, so of course when they told me it was cancer – oh, I cried and I said it's history repeating itself. Mum went down to about 4 stone, she was like a little doll lying on the settee and I said there's no way my kids are going to see me get like that and I said I was going to take a lot of tablets.

> We're not lucky people in our family – my Dad died of lung cancer and my Mum with breast cancer. I know I'm going to go that way too.

Not surprisingly, some women with breast cancer become extremely anxious about their daughters and their granddaughters and those women who do have a daughter who develops the disease may become overwhelmed with guilt about the fact that they 'passed it on'. Such women need skilled counselling and those women who are at increased risk due to heredity factors should also be counselled and screened regularly.

Divine retribution

If women can find some cause for their breast cancer it does provide a limited illusion of control over what happens to them in the future, even if this means that they themselves assumed 'responsibility' for the disease. This self-blame can be maladaptive and produce guilt about things which may have happened in the past. For example, it is not uncommon for women (especially since the revelations about cervical cancer) to feel that cancer is their 'punishment' for various real or imagined sexual improprieties.

> When I found the lump I knew exactly what it was and I thought this is my punishment at last for what I did. You see I had an illegitimate baby when I was 19 and I kept her. You didn't do things like that in my day, although it seems alright to be an unmarried mother nowadays. Anyway, I've always lied and told everyone that my husband was dead.

> This is God's punishment for my wickedness. I had an affair once with a married man. I'd always had large breasts and that's what attracted him I suppose.

Lifestyle and guilt

> *Patient:* I do blame myself in some ways for getting it, although I know now that my whole history and background and so on meant that I was almost *bound* to get it, you know, my mother having it, and putting on a lot of weight and not having much self-esteem and all that sort of thing.... I really think that worrying about it and thinking about it and being conscious of it, that is a contributory factor too.
>
> *Interviewer:* So that's the bit that you really feel guilty about?
>
> *Patient:* Yes, because I really feel that with this Bristol programme... if people can sort of visualize their tumours in such a way that they can destroy them or reduce them, so the reverse is true too. I really do believe that, you know, I was often thinking obsessively about my mother and that sort of thing being the same age and I think it all combined with my psychological make-up in the development [of the cancer].

There is a current vogue for various alternative cancer 'treatments' that employ dietary and various psychological regimens such as imagery, imaging, and assertiveness. Most of these therapies are based on the notion that people have caused their own cancer by being either too emotional, too repressed, or too stressed or have committed various dietary indiscretions. Although the contribution of any of these psychosocial factors is likely to be small and less significant than, for example, hereditary factors, individuals are encouraged to take responsibility for their cure with programmes of dietary and spiritual self-help. This form of 'treatment' will be discussed more fully in Chapter 5, but the obvious implication, that if you can cure yourself by these means then you probably caused the cancer in the first place by your faulty life-style or personality, may induce considerable guilt and distress. A failure to obtain objective improvement from such treatments can be seen as 'not fighting hard enough' or not sticking to the diet, all of which can compound further the guilt at having caused the cancer in the first place.

Stress

> I firmly believe it was the car accident and the shock that could have done it.

> Well I think it's obvious what caused it don't you – my son, my only son was murdered in Greece. We were on holiday there, my husband and I, and persuaded him to come and join us. If I hadn't begged him to come, he would still be alive. I'll never forgive myself and I'll never get over the shock of it all. We were both under a lot of stress, what with the police investigation and all. Now my husband's got heart trouble and I've got this breast thing.

There have been innumerable other anecdotal observations suggesting that exposure to stressful events is a precursor to the development of cancer. Sir James Paget, a nineteenth-century pathologist, claimed that 'deep anxiety, deferred hope and disappointment are quickly followed by the growth and increase of cancer'. It was Snow who attempted the first statistical study of women with breast cancer in 1893. He found that in 156 of 250 women who presented with either uterine or breast cancer 'there had been immediately antecedent trouble, often in very poignant form such as the loss of a near relative'.

Despite these early observations and the readiness of patients to attribute their cancer to 'stress', there is still somewhat equivocal evidence from controlled studies. Some studies show no or even negative correlations between stressful events and breast cancer. Schonfield (1975), for example, measured the number of stressful life events reported by 112 women prior to breast biopsy and found a significantly higher incidence of events in those women with benign breast lumps rather that those later found to have malignant disease. Another study by Priestman *et al.* (1985) reported that exposure to stressful life events was higher in 100 control subjects than in 100 women with benign breast disease and another 100 women with breast cancer. Ewertz (1986) looked for an association between bereavement and breast cancer in 3,520 Danish women and found no significant differences between married women and widows in terms of breast cancer risk.

Other studies do provide some support for the early anecdotal observations, for example Cooper *et al.* (1989) examined the incidence and perception of psychosocial stress amongst 1,596 symptomatic patients presenting at breast clinics and 567 attending a Well-Woman clinic for a routine medical check-up. They found some evidence that certain life events, such as death of a husband or close friend, was significantly related to breast disease (but not necessarily breast cancer). The most important finding from this study was that women found to have breast cancer *perceive* the impact of various life events as having had a severe effect. In other words, it may not be noxious life events in themselves that act as a precursor to breast cancer so much as the meaning that these life events have for individuals. These issues will be discussed further in Chapter 5, but in summary, a recent review by Hu and Silberfarb (1988) found seven studies showing a positive correlation between loss of an important other, increased life stress, and the development of cancer, and nine studies showing a negative correlation. Little has changed since Peters and Mason's review (1979) which concluded that 'experimental support can be found for essentially any view concerning the influence of stress on neoplasia'.

Personality

It is possible that personality factors or behaviour characteristics might well prove to be more salient predictors or precursors to breast cancer than stress-inducing life events. Grossarth-Maticek *et al.* (1989), for example, reported an interesting study conducted on two culturally different populations in Yugoslavia and in West Germany. They identified, via a specially constructed questionnaire, four types of behaviour patterns linked to specific types of stress and reactions to stress. Type I was characterized by

a strong need to be close to some emotionally important person or to achieve some important goal. The object, however, has withdrawn permanently and become unobtainable. Nevertheless, it continues to be perceived as the most important condition of one's well-being. Attempts to find an object that may replace it, or at least disengage emotionally from it, have failed altogether. On the contrary, the object is more or less idealised, while the self is more or less down-graded. What ensues is depression and hopelessness (which, however, the subject tries to conceal) and even a desire for death (but suicide is excluded out of sense of duty, regard for family, etc.).

In their study Grossarth-Maticek *et al.* found cancer mortality was two to five times the average in those people classified as belonging to Type I. On a more positive note, these researchers provided evidence that prophylactic interventions aimed at modifying the Type I behaviour produced a substantial reduction in cancer mortality. This is potentially very important, as health carers are by and large unable to influence the 'buffets of ill-fortune' which occur to people in 'the passage through life', but we can identify personality characteristics which may well place people at risk of developing breast cancer and offer cognitive behaviour therapies that may help.

Examples of Type I behaviour can be seen retrospectively in some of the following quotations taken from our own study:

> Quite honestly I wasn't really bothered when he said I'd got breast cancer – my life ended with G's death. He was my whole world. Without him I only exist. The past 2 years have been terrible – the only reason for living now is the dog. I take her for a walk to the cemetery every day and we talk to G. When she goes, there won't be much point in going on – she's my only link with G that's left.

Doubtless the recent publicity given to the notion that personality factors may exert a small influence on the development of breast cancer will mean that future populations of women sampled about causal factors will include personality type.

Implications of beliefs

To health care professionals some of the lay beliefs about causal factors in breast cancer may appear irrational or implausible. However, for an individual, finding a cause for disease or the presence of a symptom is extremely important, as it can be psychologically very damaging to feel that things just happen to one with no apparent explanation. The sudden appearance of a cancer produces the need to rationalize its presence by attribution of a tangible and understandable cause such as a bump or an infection. This 'effort after meaning' is seen in many other illnesses, and fulfils the important psychological need to make sense of a situation and regain mastery and control.

It is extremely important that efforts are made to understand the kinds of attitudes and beliefs that women have about breast cancer and its causal factors as they have implications for all stages of the management of the disease. A general understanding of lay beliefs may not be sufficient as some health beliefs and attitudes may be very disease specific. For example, an interesting study by Kroode *et al.* (1989) compared the causal attributions of cancer patients with those of patients who had experienced a heart attack. The major finding was that the cardiac patients looked in their past histories for causes that correlated with medical opinion, whilst the cancer patients attributed their disease to very personal, idiosyncratic causes which bore little relationship to the causal factors expressed by their relatives or their physicians. Studies such as this are extremely important for everyone involved in attempts to help patients cope with their disease and treatment. Furthermore, they are also important for all those engaged in designing health promotion campaigns to encourage the uptake of screening and breast self-examination.

Mammographic screening and breast self-examination

Utilization of screening

The various hypotheses women have concerning the causal factors in breast cancer doubtless influence their own perceived susceptibility to the disease and may therefore affect their health behaviour. Several studies have shown that a belief of personal susceptibility to breast cancer is a powerful motivator to attend for screening, e.g., Hobbs *et al.* (1980), Morris and Greer (1982), and Rutledge *et al.* (1988). However, susceptibility is not the sole criterion predicting willingness to accept breast cancer screening; other criteria are shown in Table 2.2. The health belief model of Rosenstock (1974), for example, would suggest that for a woman to engage in such things as breast self-examination (BSE) or to go along for mammographic screening she must:

Perceive herself as susceptible to the disease.

Perceive the seriousness of breast cancer and appreciate that it would have an impact on some component of life.

Feel that the treatments offered are efficacious and that early detection would reduce the severity of the disease.

Believe that the disease could be present without overt symptoms.

27

Table 2.2 Application of Rosenstock's health belief model (1974) to breast cancer screening

1	Belief in personal susceptibility to breast cancer
2	Belief that breast cancer would have at least a moderately severe impact on some component of life
3	Belief that attending for mammographic screening would have beneficial impact, i.e., early detection would reduce severity of disease
4	Belief that disease can be present without experiencing symptoms
5	Belief in the efficacy of treatments
6	Belief that the potential benefits outweigh the costs

Calnan's review (1984) of the health belief model as it applies to breast cancer and participation in programmes for early detection argued that health belief variables exerted a small impact, but that they were the best discriminators in the take up of screening.

The health beliefs held by women are developed and maintained by a large number of both external and internal factors; merely improving knowledge and education about breast cancer is unlikely to promote active participation in screening services. The normative, cultural values of an individual, together with the social influence, behaviour, and beliefs of family, friends, and important others may act as either major barriers or triggers to the acceptance of all sorts of preventative health measures including screening (Fishbein and Ajzen 1975; Hobbs *et al.* 1977). Thus, apparently conflicting beliefs and behaviours can only be understood when set in their wider complex psychological and social context. A woman may well appreciate the seriousness of breast cancer, for example, and that she herself is susceptible to the disease, all of which might predict a high 'readiness to take action', i.e., to go along for screening. However, negative aspects of the action may well prevent positive action from taking place; for example, extreme embarrassment at revealing the breasts or unwillingness to lose payment by taking time off work. Such problems can be seen in Stillman's study (1977) which looked at health beliefs and breast self-examination. She reported that embarrassment was a strong factor in deterring women from practising BSE *despite* their belief in high susceptibility to the disease.

Some women decline the offer of mammographic screening as acceptance makes them confront anxiety-provoking beliefs about breast cancer or makes them aware of inconsistencies between their beliefs and those of others. An example of this can be seen in the following quotation from a woman who refused to attend the breast screening clinic in SE London.

> I really don't want to know if I have cancer, it cannot be cured, so I prefer to remain as I am, daft as it may sound to you.

Although this woman was aware of her susceptibility to the disease and the seriousness of it, her belief that treatment was ineffective prevented her from accepting screening. Furthermore, she was obviously aware that her decision was inconsistent with others and might sound 'daft'. Women who do not believe in the efficacy of treatment will not be motivated to participate in schemes aimed at early detection of disease. Another woman, who also rejected screening, refused to complete any questionnaires designed to elicit information about health beliefs and knowledge of breast cancer. She wrote over the questionnaires:

> I have no beliefs in any of the following. I have never seriously considered the problem.

Whilst such an apparently complacent attitude might truly reflect the woman's feelings, it is more likely that she preferred to avoid the anxiety engendered by acknowledging such things as her own vulnerability to breast cancer. Attending screening or even filling in a questionnaire about breast cancer demands that fears and anxiety about the disease are confronted. McEwen et al. (1989) found that fear of cancer or preferring not to know was one of the primary reasons given for non-attendance in the SE London screening clinic by 21 per cent of the 34 women interviewed in their study.

Fink et al. (1968) suggested that women with these attitudes probably form a 'hard core' of women unlikely to ever participate in screening programmes. More recent work by French et al. (1982) highlighted this difficulty in their study of attendance at a breast-screening clinic in Edinburgh. Despite the fact that both attenders and non-attenders expressed equal knowledge about breast cancer and its treatment, there were obvious differences in attitudes, which led the authors to conclude that there is 'an important irreducible element to non-attendance due to attitudinal factors'. Twice as many non-attenders as attenders felt fearful of cancer being found and 72 per cent of non-attenders in comparison to 13 per cent of attenders felt anxious at the disruption to their lives

29

if cancer were found. The women with these negative attitudes saw a breast-screening clinic as 'a place of risk' and felt that it was better not to go looking for trouble. Many of these women rationalized their non-attendance by exaggerating the difficulties of home and work commitments. In fact, the attenders had greater occupational and domestic commitments, but nevertheless changed appointments or made arrangements to attend.

The National Breast Screening Programme which commenced in 1988 following the acceptance by the DHSS of the Forrest Report, recommended that all women between the ages of 50 and 65 years be screened every 3 years. Such a time interval means that breast self-examination may have a significant role to play in early detection. (In many parts of the world mammographic screening will *never* be a feasible proposition.) Furthermore, those women under the age of 50 or over the age of 65 should know how to examine their breasts properly. Provided that women do perform BSE effectively, there is some evidence to show that it is worthwhile. Foster and Costanza (1984) looked at 1,004 women and found that BSE was positively associated with earlier clinical stage, smaller tumours, fewer axillary nodes and significantly increased survival. More recently, Mant *et al.* (1987) found that lumps detected by women practising BSE were generally smaller than those discovered by chance. However, there are many psychosocial barriers to the practice of BSE.

Characteristics of women who practise BSE

Table 2.3 provides a summary of the psychological and social characteristics of women who engage in BSE, although it is worth pointing out that few women do examine their breasts regularly, if at all. Most authorities suggest that monthly BSE is appropriate, but there is not any evidence about the advantages of this arbitrarily chosen frequency. One of the characteristics of women who practise BSE regularly, especially if they are under 35 years, is the finding that they also engage in many other preventative health behaviours, such as dental check-ups and cervical screening (Turnbull 1798; MacLean *et al.* 1984). Other researchers have pointed out that for middle-aged women, who are more at risk from breast cancer, social class is the most pertinent factor distinguishing between acceptors and non-acceptors of preventative behaviour (Calnan 1985). Stillman (1977) reported that 40 per cent of American women practised BSE at least

Table 2.3 Characteristics of women who practise BSE

1	Engage in other preventive health measures, e.g., cervical smears, dental check-ups, etc.
	(Turnbull 1978)
2	Feel that breast cancer is the worst imaginable disease to affect women.
	(Hobbs *et al.* 1981)
3	Feel confident that they are good at performing self-examination.
	(Smith *et al.* 1980)
4	Are optimistic about likelihood of cure if treatment given at early stage.
	(Hobbs *et al.* 1981)
5	Are better educated, younger, and belong to higher socioeconomic groups than non-examiners.
	(Calnan *et al.* 1983)

monthly, but these women were mainly well-educated 35 to 50 year olds.

In Britain, estimates of the numbers of women who claim to practise BSE regularly vary from 20 per cent (Duffy and Owens 1984) to 3 per cent (MacLean *et al.* 1984). There are a variety of reasons why the majority of women fail to practise BSE despite their having adequate knowledge about breast cancer and accurate perceptions of susceptibility and seriousness. For example, some women find BSE embarrassing and there are reports that differences exist between different religious groups (Gold 1964).

An example of embarrassment about touching the breasts can be seen in this extract from an interview I had with a 60-year-old woman with breast cancer. Her cancer, which was advanced, had been detected in casualty, where she had been taken with a broken hip following a fall.

Interviewer: So the breast lump was really quite big when the doctor found it?

Patient: Yes, I suppose it was.

Interviewer: Were you aware that you had a lump there at all?

Patient: No, I wasn't.

Interviewer: Were you in the habit of checking your breasts for lumps at all?

Patient: No, never, I wasn't brought up to do that sort of thing.

Interviewer: I'm sorry to press you, but could you explain what you mean by that?

Table 2.4 Characteristics of women who attend breast-screening clinics

1	More likely to practise BSE regularly.
	(Calnan *et al.* 1983)
2	Are younger, more affluent, and of higher socioeconomic status than non-attenders.
	(Rutledge *et al.* 1988)
3	Tend to see themselves as healthy.
	(Calnan 1985)
4	Have a better knowledge of breast cancer
	(Rutledge *et al.* 1988)
5	Perceive themselves to be susceptible to breast cancer.
	(Rutledge *et al.* 1988)
6	Perceive the benefits of screening.
	(Rutledge *et al.* 1988)

Patient: We were very committed church-goers in my family. We were brought up very strictly. Touching your own body is sinful. We didn't even have mirrors in the house. I've never seen myself completely unclothed. I'm embarrassed by nakedness.

This extract represents a rather extreme view, but it is very common for women, particularly the more elderly women, to express the opinion that breast self-examination is a somewhat vulgar or risqué behaviour!

Another factor militating against BSE is linked with the suggested frequency of a month, which may well be too long a time interval for the behaviour to develop into an automatic habit. Finally, looked at from a behavioural viewpoint, BSE is not 'rewarding' in the sense that finding a lump is 'punished' and failure to find a lump provides no 'reinforcement'.

Characteristics of women who attend breast-screening clinics

The characteristics of women who are more likely to accept invitations for breast cancer screening identified in various studies are shown in Table 2.4. This shows that an important predictor of attendance is social class and several writers have pointed out that acceptors of breast cancer screening, are like acceptors of BSE, younger and of higher socioeconomic status than non-acceptors (Morris and Greer 1982; Chamberlain *et al.* 1975; Rutledge *et al.*

1988, Hunt *et al.* 1988; Owens *et al.* 1987). The fact that women less than 50 years old are more likely to accept breast cancer screening is a problem as it is the *older* woman who is most at risk from breast cancer and therefore the over 50s are the population most likely to benefit from early detection by mammography.

Conclusions

Exhortations by health educationists and credible others may well be successful in persuading women of the benefits of practising BSE regularly or in attending for mammographic screening, but this does not necessarily lead to compliance. The other competing attitudes and psychosocial factors influential in women's lives may be more persuasive and lead to rejection of the early detection procedures. The delicate balancing of the message which aims to elevate anxiety sufficiently to make them realize the seriousness of breast cancer and in so doing motivate them to participate in screening programmes, without provoking paralysing fear of the disease or inducing hyper-vigilant monitoring and obsessional examination of the breasts, is very difficult to achieve. Furthermore, until we have more reliable evidence that the treatment of the small screen-detected lesions picked up by mammography is both necessary and effective, no woman should be repeatedly cajoled into accepting screening. It is salutary to remember that mammographic screening is not so much a preventative measure as an early detection procedure. In the words of Maureen Roberts, the clinical director of the Edinburgh Breast Screening Project, who herself died of breast cancer in 1989:

it is difficult to know how to propose a health education programme for women, but the currently expressed or strongly implied statement that if women attend for screening everything will be all right is not acceptable.

For an individual woman, given her own social circumstances and particular attitudes and beliefs, non-attendance at a screening centre may well be a rational decision.

Chapter three

Finding a breast lump and hearing the diagnosis

Finding a breast lump

I was turning over in bed and I thought oh no – I knew exactly what it was. I woke up my husband and I said to him 'I've got cancer'.

I was having a bath and I felt the lump. I felt sick and shook all over – my Mum died of breast cancer, so I guessed straight away what it was.

Well I was sitting down knitting actually and the end of the needle dug my breast when I leaned over to pick up some more wool. I rubbed it and noticed the lump. I got up and looked in the mirror and saw a sort of dent, but I thought that might have been the knitting needle. It was still there in the morning, so I phoned my daughter-in-law – she used to be a nurse. She came round and marched me straight down to the doctors.

Most women realize the significance of their symptoms straightaway, although a surprisingly high number delay consulting a doctor about their breast lump. Knopf (1974) found that 80 per cent of the general public knew that the presence of a breast lump could mean cancer. In the past fifteen years, breast cancer has received so much publicity on the radio and television and there has been such a vast number of articles written in newspapers and magazines about the subject, that it would be rather difficult not to realize the potential significance of a breast lump. However, as I mentioned in the last chapter, lay populations consistently overestimate the mortality figures for cancer in all sites, and they underestimate the survival rates. Hence, many women suffer extreme anxiety and pessimism on finding a lump, which leads to considerable mental and social dysfunction. This fear of breast cancer can also lead to delay in reporting suspicious symptoms.

Delay in reporting a breast lump

One of the most frequently used coping strategies in everyday life is denial and this is also a common reaction employed by women who discover a breast lump. Denial can be seen in the following passage from an interview I conducted with a woman who was subsequently found to have a large, central malignant tumour that necessitated treatment by mastectomy:

Interviewer: What did you think that the lump was when you found it?

Patient: Well, I tried not to think about it. I didn't say anything to anyone 'cause I had the family here and I thought, oh, dear, this will spoil everyone's Christmas. But I was frightened, very frightened, but I mean you can't ignore it can you? Each morning when I got up I thought it won't be there, it won't be there, it's just imagination – but it was still there.

Whilst denial, following the discovery of a breast lump, can be a protective mechanism from a psychological point of view, paradoxically it can be a biologically damaging strategy to pursue. Although complete denial is a somewhat rare situation, some women fail to seek advice about breast lumps, convincing themselves that it is just a pulled muscle or a swollen gland until the really unpleasant symptoms of advanced cancer become impossible to disregard. Sadly, these cases are then very difficult to treat and survival may have been compromised. Sometimes the word denial is used to describe a much more frequent occurrence, that of suppression, where women attempt to conceal or suppress the fact that they have a breast lump in an attempt to avoid upsetting themselves and their families. The quotation above is probably a better example of suppression/denial than frank denial. Suppressors also tend to rationalize their delay by seeking out 'good' reasons or excuses for not seeking medical attention.

Interviewer:	How long did you wait between finding the lump and going to your GP?
Patient:	Well remember I told you that at first I thought it was just a pulled muscle – nothing to worry about really.
Interviewer:	How long did you have this pulled muscle for then?
Patient:	Well about 3–4 months I suppose.
Interviewer:	Then what happened?
Patient:	Well I still didn't think much of it – I was so busy you see, what with my daughter getting married and everything. We had relatives coming over from Australia to stay and I had to get the bedroom redecorated for them. So what with one thing and another I didn't have much time to go to the doctors did I?
Interviewer:	So what finally made you go?
Patient:	My nipple went in and I could feel a definite lump and as I had to go for my husband's prescription anyway I thought I'd mention it.
Interviewer:	So how long was it from the 'pulled muscle' to you eventually seeing the doctor?
Patient:	Well, let me see, about 9 months I suppose, but I couldn't really have gone any sooner could I? I sensed that he was rather cross with me, so was the doctor at the hospital. They never understand the work we women have to do for a wedding. That's men for you!

Can we identify any key characteristics of women who delay seeking treatment? In an important study, reported twenty-five years ago by Aiken-Swan and Paterson (1955), of women who delayed, two groups of patients were identified: those few women who were quite genuinely ignorant of the sinister implications of their symptoms and another group who understood the symptoms but were characterized by their overwhelming fear of doctors, hospitals, illness in general, and cancer in particular. The key variables found in other studies comparing the psychosocial character of delayers and non-delayers are summarized in Table 3.1. Several studies report that delayers are generally older women of lower socioeconomic class who are less well educated than non-delayers (Cameron and Hinton 1968; Greer 1974; Williams *et al.* 1976).

Table 3.1 Characteristics of women likely to delay reporting a breast lump

1	Older
2	Less likely to seek help with *any* physical symptom
3	Lower social class
4	Less well-educated
5	Habitual deniers in crises
6	More depressed
7	More anxious
8	More pessimistic about treatment
9	Fearful of surgery
10	Fearful of cancer
11	Well-defined 'body-boundaries'
12	More inhibited
13	Ignorance of significance of symptoms

To a certain extent these factors may explain delay due to ignorance of the significance of symptoms. Women from lower socio-economic groups tend to be less likely to seek help with any physical symptom. Another interesting characteristic of women who delay reporting a breast lump is that they tend to be those who habitually respond with denial to any life crisis (Greer 1974). Evidence of anxiety and a general pessimism about the efficacy of treatment is also apparent in those who delay (Gold 1964; Cameron and Hinton 1968; Margarey *et al.* 1977), although high anxiety and fear of cancer can also motivate prompt consultation (Eardley and Wakefield 1976). One problem with many of the studies examining delay is the fact that they tend to be retrospective. Consequently, the personality characteristics found could be explained by such things as guilt, the need to rationalize, embarrassment at having behaved 'stupidly' or fear that delay may have caused a poorer prognosis. A good review of the data and discussion about the methodological constraints of interpretation can be found in Ray and Baum (1985).

Some workers have estimated that approximately 20 per cent of women with symptoms of breast cancer delay seeking advice for three months or more (Cameron and Hinton 1968; Williams *et al.* 1976). Ellman (1989) has suggested that delay amongst British women in consulting about breast lumps might well be contributing to the uncomfortably high mortality rate in Great Britain.

One further point about delay in reporting the presence of a breast lump, which demonstrates that lack of knowledge is not necessarily the primary barrier, was made in an interesting study reported by Buttlar and Templeton (1983). They looked at delay and the size of breast lumps in female health care professionals and found that this group of women, especially the nurses, reported their lumps later and generally had larger tumours than other groups of women. Clearly an excess of knowledge about breast cancer and its treatment can inhibit health carers from seeking advice at an appropriate time. The behaviours may be due to anxiety, denial, or a supreme sense of complacency of the 'it couldn't happen to me' variety. This is an area of research that needs more work.

Waiting for the results

> It was a living nightmare, that three weeks – knowing what it was but not knowing for sure. Nothing that has happened since – the mastectomy or the [radiotherapy] treatment sessions were as bad as that time. Thinking it might be cancer and it spreading everywhere was all that I could do night and day.

As the quotation above aptly demonstrates, many women state that the time between finding a breast lump and having a diagnosis of cancer confirmed is the most psychologically stressful part of the whole experience (Maguire 1976, Fallowfield et al. 1987). Maguire reported that only 8 per cent of his sample of women claimed not to have been extremely concerned.

In one study done by Scott (1983), anxiety and cognitive functioning were measured in eighty-five women awaiting breast biopsy and then again six weeks later when the biopsies had confirmed benign breast disease. Prior to biopsy, she reported severe impairment of critical thinking and concentration, together with elevated anxiety rates; comparative assessments made six to eight weeks after the biopsy showed that cognitive ability had improved and anxiety levels had normalized. Early studies, such as the seminal work by Renneker and Cutler (1952), suggested that fear of losing the breast was the primary reason for distress but much of the work done more recently has shown that fear of cancer rather than surgery is the reason for the high levels of anxiety in most women. Fallowfield et al. (1990) found that only 12 per cent of their sample of 269 gave breast loss as their primary focus of concern with 59 per cent more distressed at the prospect of having cancer.

Personality and coping styles on hearing the diagnosis

The manner in which different women respond to the diagnosis of breast cancer varies enormously. These variations may be due to such things as individual coping strategies and personality factors, the level of social support available to help sustain a woman through her ordeal, and to a large extent the consultation skills of her medical carers, especially the surgeon who breaks the bad news. Before reaching the surgeon's clinic most women have mentally rehearsed the possibility that their symptoms might mean cancer and many may have imagined all sorts of depressing scenarios, especially the need for mutilating surgery followed by a painful, lonely, and undignified death.

> I went through hell, back and beyond that fortnight before I saw Mr C. I imagined the worst – no chest, no hair and dying anyway.

Not surprisingly, for some women the eventual diagnosis and discussion about treatment can be viewed as a relief. When some of the uncertainty is dissipated, it allows patients to embark on the important process of adjusting and coping.

> When he said, 'The tests show that it's cancer', I was actually quite relieved. It might sound silly, but at last someone had told me and I could stop worrying about what it might be. I couldn't wait to have the operation and start living again. I slept for the first time in two weeks that night.

The provision of clear, accurate information given in a sensitive and unhurried manner can greatly enhance the ability of a woman to take in the news and find something more positive and hopeful to help her.

However, not all women experience this sense of relief. Some react with extreme tearfulness, anger or horror.

> I'll never forget that moment – it was quite dreadful. He only got as far as saying 'I'm very sorry to have to tell you this...' and I just collapsed in floods of tears.

> When he said that awful word cancer, I just felt so angry. I was angry with everyone: my GP [General Practitioner] who told me that I didn't have to worry, it wouldn't be cancer; with the nurse in the clinic, who was being so nice; with God; with the whole

world. I kept screaming, it's not fair, why me, what have I ever done to deserve this? Poor man, he looked shell-shocked when I left the clinic.

Some women experience an extreme sense of shock when they hear the diagnosis. These are usually patients who are genuinely unaware of the seriousness of their symptoms and are therefore unprepared for the bad news, or they are women who have successfully employed denial, but suddenly find themselves being forced to confront the reality of malignant disease.

It came as a total shock. I was absolutely stunned. All the time I'd thought that it was going to be a cyst.

I felt as though someone had quite literally punched me. I was completely stunned. All the time I'd been telling myself that it was just my imagination, that there wasn't really anything wrong – some people are just a bit lumpy. The shock was indescribable.

Other women immediately think of the impact that breast cancer and its treatment might have on their relationships with family and friends.

My husband was holding my hand when Mr P. told me and I felt him flinch. Then I thought, 'Oh, my God, he won't ever want to touch me again'. I felt so dirty and unclean.

All I kept thinking was 'what am I going to tell my family?'. We're very close you know, but not very good about personal things to do with illness. We don't talk about cancer and switch programmes about hospitals or starving children off.

I immediately thought of my poor husband – he's bed-ridden with a bad heart and has had a stroke. I'm all he's got and I dread to think what would happen to him without me. I didn't know how I was going to tell him, as the shock could have killed him. Mr H. was so kind and understanding and didn't mind when I shed a tear.

It has been suggested that there are clearly identifiable categories of response to the diagnosis of breast cancer. Morris and her colleagues (1977) outlined five: denial, fighting spirit, stoic acceptance, anxious/depressed acceptance, and helpless/hopelessness. Although these last two categories were added together in later work by Morris and her colleagues, we have found examples of all five responses amongst our own patients, some of which are given below.

Denial

I have already described how some women cope with the discovery of a breast lump by denial. Likewise, this strategy may also be employed when the doctor imparts the diagnosis. The women reject the seriousness of the evidence offered to them and appear reluctant to engage in any detailed discussion of the subject.

> They told me before that it was just mastitis, so I tried to think that was all it was again. I'm not the sort of person to ask a lot. I'd rather they didn't tell me.

> Well I don't think that these experts always know what's going on and just to be on the safe side they prefer to treat breast lumps as serious just in case.

Fighting spirit

Women who fell into this category were those who displayed a positive, hopeful approach to the news and who tended to solicit as much information as possible about their diagnosis and treatment.

> I'm not giving in, whatever happens. I'm going to fight this thing.

> I just said to him I want the truth with no frills and I want whatever treatment will help me survive this thing.

> As soon as I knew for sure, I read everything I could about the subject. I never really thought about dying. I was only interested in how I could keep living.

Stoic acceptance

Morris *et al.* reported that more than half of their sample of women reacted in this way and furthermore that this coping strategy was maintained throughout their illness. Stoic acceptors display quiet acknowledgement of the diagnosis and a philosophical or phlegmatic approach to their future treatment and whatever lies ahead.

> I knew what he was going to say. I was quite prepared. I know

that it's out of my hands – what will be, will be. It's pointless worrying.

Well I didn't cry or anything, I just accepted it. I'm a Christian you see and I believe that whatever happens is God's will.

Anxious/depressed acceptance

Some women react with excessive anxiety and/or depression. They tend to regard all the comments made about their diagnosis and treatment with pessimism, but nevertheless find some means of continuing with their usual activities.

I didn't take any time off work; I had to keep going. The trouble was every time I took an order or arranged a meeting I kept thinking 'I might not be around for it'. Everything I did seemed rather pointless. I was sure that I wasn't going to be one of the lucky ones.

I don't know how I'd have got through that week if I hadn't been so busy with the children; but then they made it worse too. I kept thinking 'God, they're going to be orphans'.

Helpless/hopelessness

Arguably the most difficult group of women to help in any way are those who become so totally engulfed with a sense of helplessness and hopelessness when they hear their diagnosis that they view the future with extreme pessimism and exhibit high levels of social dysfunction. These women are incapable of seeing themselves as anything other than actively ill or dying.

We're not lucky people in our family – my Dad died of cancer, and my Mum. I know I'm going to go that way too. The only thing I like is my garden, but I haven't planted any bulbs even – what's the point? I won't see them will I?

The doctor's role in ameliorating the impact of 'bad news'

Some of the important issues and implications that a knowledge of the responses described above has for effective doctor/patient communication will be discussed further in Chapter 7, but there is some evidence that the skilled doctor can do a great deal to ameliorate or even prevent some of the emotional trauma provoked by the 'bad news'. The unskilled, uncaring doctor can make a difficult, sorry situation even worse for his or her unfortunate patient. Below is a passage from an article written by a woman with gyneacological cancer.

> We are all easily intimidated by a system that discourages communication, sensitivity and mutual respect. When patients are nervous to start with, a system that requires them to be stripped and lined up in examination rooms only makes matters worse. A few of the doctors I have met had sufficient empathy and interpersonal skills to overcome the communication barriers inherent in such a set up. When the doctor's manner is brusque or hurried and information given reluctantly, patients can become completely demoralised. I speak from experience.
>
> (Morton 1987)

Although this extract came from a patient who had gyneacological cancer, it is applicable to all doctors breaking bad news in any speciality. The quotation which follows comes from a 45-year-old woman with breast cancer and provides an example of an appalling lack of insight and sensitivity on the part of her surgeon.

> I felt terrible; I was scared stiff and shaky and really embarrassed lying there on the examination couch with just this flimsy gown that didn't cover me right up. He came in with a couple of young doctors, and oh I was so ashamed, the way he examined me – I've got such big breasts you see. He just didn't seem to act as though I was there and kept talking to the others about the difficulty in knowing what to do with big breasts. I asked him what was wrong with me. He said 'You must realise it's cancer; we'll have you in next week sometime' and walked out. I've never felt so confused in my life I was terrified – I'd got cancer, I didn't know what they were going to do for it, I was angry, embarrassed and didn't know what on earth to do.

This woman had recently been bereaved, her husband having died from a heart attack two months previously, and her son had been sent to prison for fraud. She was living alone in a town that she barely knew (she had only lived there for six months prior to her husband's death). Her sense of humiliation, fear, and confusion was not helped by the fact that she had no one with whom she could share her distress when she got home. Whilst the surgeon could perhaps, if one was feeling generous, be forgiven for not making time or an attempt to discover this patient's sorry social circumstances, he deserves to be castigated for the lack of respect shown her as a person. No one should be told that they have cancer without even the dignity of clothing. Neither should we tolerate any system which permits someone to be told such news with such a lack of human compassion. A hand to hold and a shoulder to cry on seem rather basic and obvious requirements for someone who had just received a diagnosis of breast cancer.

Fortunately, not all breast cancer surgeons behave in such a crass manner, as the following account shows.

> I can't speak highly enough of Mr C. He was very gentle and kind and didn't hurry me even though it was a busy clinic with lots waiting. He let me get dressed, then he sat me down, held my hand and asked me what I thought was wrong. When I said 'cancer', he said that I was right, but that I shouldn't feel too worried as the lump was very small and there wasn't any lumpiness under my arms, which is a good sign. When he'd let that sink in a bit he asked me if I knew about all the different treatments and explained the pros and cons. He asked me if I'd understood and whether or not I had anyone outside to take me home or if there was anyone the nurse could phone for me. He told me there was no hurry and that he'd like me to think about which treatment I wanted and to come back next week to talk again. He gave me the phone number of a nurse-counsellor and asked me to get in touch if I was worried or hadn't understood. It might seem funny, but I went out feeling really comforted and confident. He honestly seemed to care and be interested in me. I think he's a saint.

Apart from permitting the woman with breast cancer the dignity of clothing before breaking bad news and showing her some respect and compassion, there are also some other fairly simple things that may help. For example, one study (Fallowfield et al. 1987) reported the finding that the presence of a close relative or friend during the bad news consultation appeared to reduce the incidence of anxiety and/or depression measured in patients at twelve months. This could have been due to the fact that many patients were confused, uncertain, and anxious about their disease and its treatment, as the shock of learning the diagnosis prevents the assimilation of information, despite the doctor's best effort to explain fully.

> After he said 'cancer' I just didn't know what he was going on about. I was all by myself and so shocked, I just couldn't believe it. I thought it was a bit callous. He might just as well have not bothered. It just went in one ear and out the other.

The presence of a trusted ally in the form of a spouse, partner, friend, or relative may have proved useful in long-term adaptation, as this advocate might have been able to retain more of what the doctor had said. Therefore discussion of the various ramifications that the news had for the woman's future could have taken place later in a more informed way than would have been possible if the friend or relative had not been present. However, another important interpretation of the findings from this study is the fact that individuals who enjoy good quality social support in all situations are more able to cope with any life crisis.

Reactions of family and friends to diagnosis

The importance of good social support in long-term adjustment will be discussed more fully in Chapter 6, but it is appropriate here to describe some of the immediate reactions of family and friends to the news that their loved ones have breast cancer. Not all women tell their families about the discovery of a breast lump; they prefer to keep their fears to themselves and to go through all the investigations alone in order not to worry the family unnecessarily.

Interviewer: Did anyone come with you to the hospital to see Mr B?

Patient: No, I went on my own. I hadn't told anyone that I was going, as I hadn't told them about the lump even. I didn't want them to worry and I thought that it was just going to be something simple anyway.

Interviewer: So what did you tell them when you got back from the hospital?

Patient: Well – oh dear, it was awful – I didn't know how to start. They were all sitting down watching television after supper and I just blurted it out.

> Everyone was upset, especially my daughter and my husband went very quiet. He said that he felt hurt that I hadn't told him. But I didn't tell them everything at first – I couldn't say the word.
>
> *Interviewer:* What word?
>
> *Patient:* You know, what it really was – cancer. Telling them was worse than hearing it at the hospital.

This passage demonstrates a very real and underestimated problem which newly diagnosed patients experience – that of telling their loved ones the bad news. They may find the discussion painfully upsetting, either because the family react with great distress or sometimes because the news does not elicit the support that they had hoped for.

> He didn't say anything – not 'sorry' or 'you poor thing'. He didn't even ask when I was going to have the operation. He just went off to the pub as usual. We've been a bit distant for a few years now, but I thought that with something as horrible as this cancer, he'd show some feeling for me. I cried more about his thoughtlessness than about the cancer. I could cope with that, but not with the thought that he didn't care about me any more. I suppose that's why I didn't tell him – didn't want to put him to the test.

Another difficulty that women have when attempting to tell their loved ones what the doctor said is remembering and relaying accurately all the information. For many lay people the details about investigations or treatment options are difficult to recall. Ley and Spelman (1965) showed that, for patients seeing a physician in medical outpatients for the first time, approximately 40 per cent of the information had been lost by the time the patients' recall was tested 80 minutes later.

One novel method of helping patients break the bad news to their relatives and to assist in the recall of information was described by Hogbin and Fallowfield (1989). They provided forty-six patients, thirty-five of whom were women with carcinoma of the breast, with audio-tape recordings of their 'bad news' consultation to take home. These audiotapes contained an explicit statement of the diagnosis, that is, all patients were told that they had cancer. They also contained information concerning further tests such as bone scans;

descriptions of the various surgical options available were given, as were relevant details about radiotherapy and chemotherapy. Patients were all sent questionnaires which allowed the researchers to evaluate the benefits (or costs) of the exercise. The results showed that patients found their tapes extremely helpful for a wide variety of reasons. Their primary value was their usefulness in providing accurate information for family and friends, as the following quotations demonstrate.

> Your idea of the tape was brilliant, as I found I couldn't tell my family. They found it very helpful and it put their minds at rest. Your tape gave me great comfort and confidence in you.

> In my opinion, the tape is a very good idea, and I found it very helpful to sit down quietly to listen to the conversation again with my family and then talk it over.

Although Hogbin and Fallowfield made no attempt to formally test recall of information, self-report by 38 per cent of the patients suggested that the tapes contained information that they had forgotten.

> This [the tape] was a tremendous help, as it is impossible to recall everything said when one is in a state of shock.

Even those patients who claimed not to have forgotten anything found their tapes allowed them to rehearse and understand more about the medical terminology about which they often had little previous knowledge or experience.

> We think the tape is a very good idea, very helpful. Whilst I had not forgotten information, playing the tape on our own (my husband and me) helped to clarify the advice and information.

> I found the tape very helpful indeed for the reasons below: (1) it prevented me from unintentionally distorting any information I was given; (2) the calm and factual discussion is very useful to listen to again at times of panic and despair.

Some doctors do appear to act as though their patients inhabit a social vacuum. Consequently, pressing emotional and practical needs of the whole family may be overlooked. As the family have an important role to play in helping a woman to recover from both the physical and mental traumas associated with the diagnosis of breast cancer and its treatment, their support needs to be enlisted early on. Sometimes the mental anguish suffered by the healthy husband, children, siblings, and parents of a woman with breast cancer can match that experienced by the woman herself. They too feel such things as anxiety, due to fears about the operation, worries about their own reaction to her changed appearance, difficulty in knowing what to say and how to behave, and, of course, fears about their loved one undergoing an unpleasant and premature death. Some of these intense feelings of threat and helplessness experienced by other family members when a woman is diagnosed as having breast cancer have been described by Lewis *et al.* (1985). The relatives may feel guilty about their own good health or occasionally resentful about a woman, who fulfils a major role in keeping the family going, becoming ill with a life-threatening disease. The following quotation from the husband of a woman newly diagnosed probably reveals a mixture of all these feelings.

> I just can't believe it, it's so unfair. I've worked so hard all my life and things have been very, very tough at times, let me tell you. I've just taken retirement and had all these plans about things to do and places to go. What's all this mastectomy business going to mean, that's what I need to know? Will she still be able to do things afterwards? I'm not that good around the house. I've always taken care of the money side of things and she's looked after the kids and me. I need her, that's the sort of relationship we have. What will I do if I lose her? She will pull through, won't she?

There is little published empirical work examining the effects that a diagnosis of breast cancer has on the relatives of a sufferer, although depression and anxiety are known to be high amongst the relatives of patients diagnosed as having cancer in different sites (Maguire 1984; Plumb and Holland 1977). The children of women with breast cancer may exhibit various behavioural disorders including conflicts with their parents, regressive behaviour and/or acting-out (Wellisch 1979). This problem is more acute for adolescent daughters of women with breast cancer, as they tend to be relied upon more than sons. Not only do they become hostile or withdrawn in view of the fact that they are expected to offer more physical help, but they may also be burdened with extreme anxiety that they too will develop the disease. Lichtman *et al.* (1984) found evidence that at least 12 per cent of mother/child relationships significantly deteriorated following the mother's diagnosis of breast cancer.

Although there is a body of literature on talking to children about death and dying, there is surprisingly little about how to discuss a diagnosis of cancer with the children of sufferers. The absence of any sensible material led to an American woman, who went through the trauma of breast cancer, writing a useful article entitled 'Telling your kids you have cancer or any serious illness' (Frankel and Canepa, 1988). This woman's moving and lucid account of her disease and treatment is valuable reading and she highlights the problems confronting children with this quotation:

> My 17-year-old daughter said that being told about my breast cancer felt like a bad dream, 'I don't see any way I could have been told about it that would have made it any easier. The word cancer is so scary. Everyone was terrified. I was scared for my mother, for my family. I kept thinking, what if she dies? At night, I remember crying and crying because I felt I couldn't do anything to save her.'
>
> (Frankel 1988)

The needs of the family are sometimes overlooked, due to a mistaken view that a woman with breast cancer suffers more distress than her family. No matter how distraught the relatives may be it is too easy to assume that, out of concern for their relative with cancer, they will be able to keep their feelings in check and will be able to offer love, comfort, and practical support to her. An interesting study by Cassileth et al. (1985) assessed mood state in 200 patients with cancer and their next-of-kin. She found that although the patient group showed more depression and anxiety overall, there was a high correlation between scores for mood disorder amongst patient/next-of-kin pairs. In other words, if a patient with cancer was found to be depressed or anxious, then there was a very high probability that the next-of-kin would be also.

Spouses or partners of women with breast cancer may feel a considerable burden of responsibility in the successful adjustment of their partner to the fact of her disease and possibly her altered bodily appearance. There are accounts of how close couples become following the experience of breast cancer. For example, Hughes (1987) studied twenty-eight married couples following mastectomy. She reported that three of these (11 per cent) experienced marital problems post-treatment, but that the majority felt their relationships to be either the same or enhanced. In another study of the spouses of mastectomy patients reported by Sabo *et al.* (1986) the men were found to be suffering considerable emotional distress, but tended to hide this by displaying a minimizing, reassuring pose. They assumed that this would be seen as protective and supportive by their wives. Unfortunately, the women felt that their husbands were rejecting and insensitive to their feelings, all of which led to misunderstanding and a coldness in their relationship. For a good description of the sorts of problems that husbands are likely to experience see Gates (1980).

Relationships are always affected in some way by a woman's diagnosis of breast cancer. For those with fragile relationships this burden may prove to the final straw to break the camel's back; for the majority of women, however, it is a time when the commitment and love and affection of her family and friends are reaffirmed. Good information and counselling support provided at the outset, that is, at the time of diagnosis, should be made available to the person who shares the closest emotional relationship with the patient, as it is this 'most significant other' who will be one of the most important factors in a woman's long-term adjustment.

Chapter four

Psychosocial outcome of breast cancer treatment

Depression is a common sequel to mastectomy, and is marked by anxiety, insomnia, depressive attitudes, occasional ideas of suicide, and feelings of shame and worthlessness.

(Renneker and Cutler 1952)

Psychiatric morbidity

There have been many largely anecdotal descriptions of the extreme psychological distress, social, and sexual difficulties associated with breast cancer treatment. Two seminal papers published in the 1950s by Renneker and Cutler and Bard and Sutherland described the psychological sequelae following mastectomy. Their work revealed that anxiety and depression, together with impairments to physical and sexual functioning were very common features post-operatively. At the time these articles were published radical mastectomy was almost the only treatment available; an unpleasantly mutilating procedure based on the flawed premise that the more tissue that was removed the more likely the surgeon would be to extirpate all the cancer. As was shown in Chapter 1, what we now know of the biology of breast cancer does not permit any confidence in the view that the greater the mutilation the greater the chance of halting cancer spread. Consequently, many thousands of women did suffer significant psychological and physical impairments following unnecessarily radical surgery. However, it is always a salutary lesson to look at the alternative facing women and their surgeons at that time; uncontrolled breast cancer leading to a painful, odorous, fungating, broken-down chest wall is not a very pleasant sight or experience.

Table 4.1 Psychological outcome of mastectomy (Mx) vs. breast conservation (BC)

Authors	Patients	Derivation of sample	Outcome
Sanger and Reznikoff 1981	40 Mx (20) BC (20)	Diverse sources: non-comparable treatment groups.	*No difference between groups in psychosocial morbidity. Greater overall 'body satisfaction' in in BC group.*
Schain et al. 1983	38 Mx (20) BC (18)	Randomized clinical trial.	*No significant psychosocial differences, but less negative body image in BC group.*
Steinberg et al. 1985	67 radical Mx (46) BC (21) ($\frac{1}{2}$ chose BC)	Retrospective study: non-comparable treatment groups. No information on how sample was selected from those eligible.	*No significant differences between groups in psychosocial morbidity. BC group less self-conscious.*
Ashcroft et al. 1985	40 Mx? BC? (numbers unknown)	Some women randomized and some women chose treatment (numbers not given): prospective study of consecutive cases.	*Little difference between groups on psycho-social measures but better body satisfaction in BC group.*
de Haes et al. 1985	39 Mx (18) BC (21)	Randomized clinical trial. Retrospective psychological assessment.	*Less negative body image in BC group. No differences in sexual or psychological functioning or in fear of recurrence or death.*
Bartelink et al. 1985	172 Radical MX (58) BC (114)	Retrospective study of consecutive patients.	*Less negative body image and less fear of recurrence in BC group.*

Authors	Patients	Derivation of sample	Outcome
Fallowfield et al. 1986	101 Mx (53) BC (48)	Randomized clinical trial. Retrospective study.	No difference in psychiatric morbidity between groups, but more overt concern with cancer in BC group.
Lasry et al. 1987	123 Mx (43) BC+RXT (36) BC (44)	Randomized clinical trial. Retrospective study: no information on how sample was selected from those eligible.	Depression highest in BC+RXT group. Better body image in BC group. Fear of recurrence greatest amongst patients receiving chemotherapy.
Wolberg et al. 1987	206 Mx (no choice) 96 Mx (choice) 56 BC (choice) 54	Prospective study: consecutive patients.	Psychosocial data reported from only 39 eligible patients. Advantage in terms of anxiety and depression to women who chose BC.
Kemeny et al. 1988	52 Mx (27) BC (25)	Randomized clinical trial. Retrospective study.	No significant difference in psychological morbidity between groups. Less 'sadness when first viewing breast surgery' in BC group.
Morris and Royle 1988	30 Mx (no choice) 10 Mx (choice) 7 BC (choice) 13	Prospective study: consecutive patients.	No difference in psychological morbidity between Mx and BC but less morbidity in patients offered choice.
Meyer and Aspergren 1989	58 Radical Mx (30) BC (28)	Sample drawn from consecutive patients. No other details: retrospective study.	No differences in psychological morbidity between groups. Less negative body image in BC group.
Maunsell et al. 1989	227 Mx (147) BC (80)	Consecutive patients assessed at 3 and 18 months.	Significantly more psychological morbidity in BC group at 3 months. No difference at 18 months although psychological morbidity high (35%) in both.
Fallowfield et al. 1990	269 Mx (no choice) 135 3C (no choice) 72 Mx (choice) 19 3C (choice) 43	Prospective study: consecutive patients outside clinical trial setting.	No difference at 12 months in psychiatric morbidity or sexual dysfunction between 2 groups, less morbidity in patients treated by surgeons who offered choice wherever possible.

Nevertheless, radical mastectomy was a high price to pay for increased survival and many people began to question whether or not the benefits from such procedures were worth the concomitant psychological trauma. With time, fewer surgeons performed radical mastectomy and many more favoured the modified radical mastectomy or a total (simple) mastectomy, which gave a significantly more acceptable cosmetic result. However, women still lost a breast and had an unpleasant scar.

Numerous descriptions in the scientific literature and lurid accounts in the popular press continue to chart the psychosocial havoc wreaked by the diagnosis of breast cancer and its treatment, especially if that treatment involves breast amputation. Dean (1987) has estimated that the overall incidence of psychiatric morbidity following mastectomy is approximately three times that likely to be found in the general population of women. Not surprisingly, the development of breast-conserving techniques which involve excision of the malignant lump (lumpectomy) followed by radiotherapy have been supported enthusiastically by many women. Also substantial numbers of surgeons, who had always disliked performing mutilating procedures for breast cancer, have become committed advocates of breast conservation.

As the reports from randomized clinical trials comparing relapse-free intervals and survival in women treated for early breast cancer by mastectomy or lumpectomy demonstrated no differences in survival between treatment groups (Veronesi *et al.* 1981; Fisher *et al.* 1985), more surgeons felt increasingly confident about offering women breast conservation. Clinicians thought that they could provide an effective treatment which would substantially reduce psychiatric morbidity without compromising survival. Whilst intuitively plausible, there is to date little evidence to suggest that breast conservation confers on women a clean bill of psychological health. There are at least fourteen published studies comparing the psychological outcome of mastectomy versus lumpectomy and these show few substantial differences between treatments. Table 4.1 gives a summary of this research work, together with the main findings.

One of the first studies to challenge the idea that breast loss caused psychiatric morbidity was a retrospective assessment of 101 women with early breast cancer who were randomized to either mastectomy or breast conservation following informed consent. The surprise and disappointment for many was that rates of anxiety and/or depression were still high whatever the surgery given (Fallowfield *et al.* 1986). Of those women who underwent mastectomy 32 per cent were rated as anxious and/or depressed, as were 38 per cent of the women who underwent breast-conserving surgery. Some researchers suggested that these counter-intuitive data resulted from the fact that women had their treatment determined following randomization and that women able to exert more autonomy would not suffer psychological distress, especially if they could choose breast conservation. These issues of 'choice' will be discussed in more detail in Chapter 7, but a more recent prospective study by the same authors of 269 women who were treated outside the setting of a clinical trial found similarly high rates of psychiatric morbidity (Fallowfield *et al.* 1990).

Interested readers should see Hall and Fallowfield (1989) for a detailed review of the other studies comparing psychological outcome, but their primary finding was that whenever psychiatric morbidity had been assessed adequately, using validated tests on a reasonable sample of women, there was very little difference between the numbers of women found to be anxious and/or depressed whatever their primary surgical therapy. A significant minority of women with early stage breast cancer (approximately 35 per cent) develop moderate to severe anxiety and/or depression as a result of both the diagnosis and the treatment. The idea that breast loss per se causes the psychological trauma is no longer supportable. Some studies show a small advantage to women who undergo breast conservation in terms of body image, and such techniques spare women the nuisance of having to wear an external prosthesis, but as we saw in Chapter 3, most women are more concerned about having cancer than about losing a breast. The diagnosis of breast cancer, which many women regard as universally fatal, together with the worry of being stigmatized, rejected, and dying a lonely, painful, and undignified death, are issues that confront all women irrespective of their surgical treatment.

The growing recognition that women may be more, or just as, anxious about the fact of having cancer as they are about potential loss of a breast means that we should look more closely at the poor counselling provision for women who have breast-conserving surgery. Such women may have many unmet psychological needs, especially if all around them hold the mistaken view that all will be well provided women avoid mastectomy. A woman aged 50 who had undergone a lumpectomy followed by radiotherapy told me:

> What I couldn't understand was why the nurses didn't have any thought for what I was going through the night before the operation. They were all terribly concerned and kind to another lady on the ward who had to have her breast removed, but no-one came and talked to me. I was really scared, all sorts of awful things were going through my mind, but I got this feeling that I was meant to be grateful to someone that I wasn't having the breast off, so I shouldn't make a fuss.

This problem may continue throughout a woman's treatment and follow-up period and I have met many women who have had to disguise their anxiety and depression following lumpectomy, or who have been made to feel guilty about experiencing unremitting distress, as this extract from an interview illustrates.

Patient: I feel so guilty about feeling so lifeless and miserable. After all, it's not as though I had to have my breast off and they say they caught it early.

Interviewer: Have you told anyone that you feel this way?

Patient: Oh, no – I mean the family have got enough to worry about. They think that I'm marvellous, but as soon as no-one's here I just cry. They expect me to be all right now.

Interviewer: Have you mentioned this to the doctor at all?

Patient: No – it wouldn't be right, would it? He's done his best. I should be grateful. Anyway, he's always so busy.

This attitude may also be a reflection of cultural conditioning where we demand an unreasonable display of stoicism in the face of both physical and emotional pain. The anxious woman with breast cancer who has had a lumpectomy is not meant to break the rules which require her to confront disease with cheerfulness and fortitude. The role of a sick person may well be legitimate for the time when she is in hospital, but as time passes with few overt signs of physical problems, then there is an unwritten social obligation to function normally and not complain. No-one can deny that the mutilation of mastectomy causes most women considerable emotional distress, but I have argued that 'the flat chest wall "legitimises" a maintenance of the sick role, whereas having "just a little lump removed" creates the feeling that as treatment was comparatively "trivial" the woman should be grateful at retaining her breast and quickly return to normal psychological functioning. When she fails to do so, guilt ensues' (Fallowfield *et al.* 1987). She may try to repress these unacceptable emotions of misery and anxiety, and failure to do so increases feelings of worthlessness. It is hardly surprising that such women can become very depressed.

One further point worth emphasizing is that although breast-conserving procedures mean a shorter hospital stay, possibly less post-operative pain and a quicker recovery from the surgery itself, the women treated in this way almost invariably have to undergo radiotherapy and if they are pre-menopausal they may be more likely to have adjuvant cytotoxic chemotherapy. It could be these adjuvant therapies which contribute to much of the adverse psychosocial sequelae in breast cancer.

Radiotherapy

The majority of women who have a lumpectomy and some women who undergo mastectomy also have a course of external beam radiotherapy (see Chapter 1). This means daily treatment, usually for a period of six weeks. Lucas *et al.* (1987) have reported strong correlations between the amount of radiotherapy given, adverse reactions, and subsequent psychiatric morbidity, but sometimes the mere thought of such treatment is enough to create anxiety. Doctors often tell women that radiotherapy is being given to 'clear up any remaining cancer cells which may be there' or 'as an insurance policy just to be sure we've got all the cancer'. Such comments may be perceived as reassuring, but for some women they arouse doubt about the adequacy of the surgery.

> I was quite angry when he said that. I mean, I thought he'd said that having the lump removed was just as safe as having the breast off. Then all this talk about 'any remaining cells will be killed by the radiotherapy' – it really worried me. I thought I'd been tricked – I was angry and scared stiff.

Another reason that radiotherapy scares women is the apparent paradox for lay people that radiation is being given to cure cancer, although it is also known to produce cancer. Media publicity surrounding accidents at nuclear power stations, such as Three-mile

Island and Chernobyl, or the continued debate and appropriate concerns about the incidence of childhood leukaemias around areas such as Sellafield, do little to allay women's fears about radiotherapy. The fact that the staff in radiotherapy departments wear protective lead aprons and retreat behind thick concrete walls also serves to increase the anxiety of patients, especially at the beginning of treatment. The following passage comes from a moving account by a 34-year-old woman who was scared and worried that the radiation would prevent her from having children.

'Well, we don't use shielding in this treatment,' said one of the radiographers. 'I mean, if you pointed this beam at a lead apron, it would go straight through,' she explained helpfully, unwittingly adding to my fears. The first experience of radiotherapy is not a happy one. You are left alone, lying motionless in a windowless room, head on one side, arm in the air clutching a handle. The radiographers leave in haste as if running for the bunker. A droning siren sounds and a red light flashes. Two closed circuit television cameras are focused on you, one on your face: even your grief is monitored. Each dose of radiation – which lasts up to two minutes – felt like an eternity, and I often wondered if they had forgotten to switch the machine off.

Later the canned music machine was mended and thereafter I was accompanied by 'Raindrops keep falling on your head' and similarly cheerful tunes.

To me, this seemed dishonest, a pretence that all was well – like a euphemism for cancer. I had six weeks of daily treatment – Monday to Friday – and soon got used to it.

(Prior 1988)

Radiotherapy can also cause unpleasant physical side effects such as anorexia, sickness, skin irritation, and an enervating fatigue. These side effects are cumulative; thus some patients feel much worse at the end of their course of treatment than they did at the beginning. This re-awakens fears that the irradiation has been harmful. In one study, almost one-third of patients were still complaining of excessive tiredness following radiotherapy a year after their treatment (Fallowfield *et al.* 1986). In answer to the question, 'Looking back over this past year, can you pick out one period that was worse than any other?' most women said that the period between finding the lump and hearing the diagnosis was the most stressful period, closely followed by their experiences during radiotherapy.

> What I hadn't bargained on was feeling so drained of energy. They tell you that you'll probably feel tired for a few days, but this has gone on for months now. I sometimes think that the treatment did more than burn out the cancer cells – it has burnt out my strength, my soul. I feel sort of empty and exhausted the whole time.

Even the knowledge that one is having radiotherapy is sufficient to produce side effects, so more needs to be done to make it a less anxiety-provoking experience. Parsons *et al.* (1961) reported that 75 per cent of patients given sham radiotherapy complained of nausea and fatigue. The depressing environment of some of our radiotherapy departments and poorly-organized appointment systems does little to ameliorate the distress experienced by some women.

> That radiotherapy was just awful – my skin burnt and I hated not being able to wash for weeks or go out in the sun. The worst thing of all though was the place itself. You had to sit in a narrow, dark corridor in those horrid hospital gowns waiting for your turn. It felt like waiting to be executed. I used to cry when I got home and have nightmares about it, especially remembering some of the other poor people there with me who were obviously dying.

This last point is worth considering a little further. As I mentioned in Chapter 3, denial is a common and important coping strategy for many women with breast cancer. Regular radiotherapy sessions waiting with other patients suffering from advanced disease make it very difficult to sustain the strategy of denial. Undoubtedly some of the anxiety and depression associated with radiotherapy is due to women being made to face the reality of their diagnosis, and seeing other seriously-ill patients can make women worry that they too will share the same fate even if they had started radiotherapy in a positive and optimistic frame of mind, as these comments from a 48-year-old woman show:

Well, I was actually rather cheerful when I first went along – the staff were all so very kind and I was really pleased that I didn't have to have a mastectomy. I was determined to be positive and keep my spirits up. There was a little boy waiting in the department with no hair, looking awful; he had a brain tumour. Three weeks later I heard that he had died. Then I got talking to another woman who had breast cancer. She'd got it back again and was coming for radiotherapy – she said it was only to stop the pain in her bones, not to try and cure her. I got terribly depressed and kept thinking why are they putting us through this if everyone ends up dying anyway?

Although I have portrayed a rather gloomy description of radiotherapy with unpleasant physical and emotional side effects, it is not a miserable experience for everyone, as this testimony from one woman demonstrates:

Oh – no, it really wasn't that bad at all – I don't know what everyone was going on about. I was a bit frightened by the machine itself at first, but you soon get used to that. I didn't have any problems with my skin and it didn't make me tired. I quite enjoyed the camaraderie; it was like being in the war. The ambulancemen who picked me up every day to take me were terrific – always joking about and so patient and kind to us all. I made some really good friends during the treatment, as you usually had to wait so long and there was plenty of time to talk. We all got very close to each other and still phone each other up. I think I was quite sad when my course of treatment finished. There were a few women who took it badly – got skin reactions and things, but we all used to try and cheer each other up. It usually helped just to share it with someone else. I was one of the lucky ones I suppose.

Another woman, far from being made anxious by the experience, felt secure and pleased that the treatment was given to 'clear up any remaining cells'.

I just used to lie there thinking of the X-rays tracking down and blasting the cancer cells. The doctor told me that the operation was the belt to hold my trousers up and the [radiotherapy] treatment the braces. I felt very certain that every bit of the cancer was being killed and that helped me through.

Chemotherapy

The experience of radiotherapy is often extremely unpleasant for many women with breast cancer, but it is not uniformly distressing and the side effects are not inevitable. In contrast, cytotoxic chemotherapy arguably has the worst reputation of all the treatments available for breast cancer, as it does produce many side effects, although they may vary in severity from individual to individual and to some extent on the drug being given and the route of administration. Most patients given cytotoxic drugs suffer from nausea, vomiting, and alopecia (hair loss). Some may also experience such things as mouth soreness, diarrhoea, and a lowering of the white cell count which reduces the resistance of the body to infection. There is some evidence that certain of the drugs used affect mood state and cognitive functioning, although these effects may be due to psychological distress as much as some direct biochemical effect on the brain (Silberfarb *et al.* 1980). Before offering cytotoxic chemotherapy very careful judgements must be made balancing side effects against potential benefits for patients with breast cancer.

The aim of all adjuvant cytotoxic therapy is to improve the likelihood of 'cure' when given immediately after local treatment for early breast cancer, or to extend survival when given to patients with advanced disease. The problem is that we have little idea as to which women will benefit from such treatment. Some patients may well go through the trauma of chemotherapy for nothing as their primary surgical therapy had been sufficient. Others may relapse with recurrent disease despite enduring the side effects of chemotherapy. Thus their sufferings will have been in vain. Research to date suggests that in early stage breast cancer there is an advantage to the pre-menopausal woman and it is this group therefore who tend to receive chemotherapy in Great Britain (Nolvadex Adjuvant Trial Organisation 1985).

For a woman who has already undergone many emotional and physical assaults, the news that she must now go through several courses of chemotherapy over a period of approximately six months is often regarded with a mixture of fear and suspicion. Just as the need for radiotherapy provokes fears that the cancer has not been removed effectively by surgery, the need for chemotherapy may create similar anxieties.

My heart sank when he said that he wanted me to have
chemotherapy. I said, wasn't it enough that he'd taken my breast
off? Surely I didn't have to go through another hell as well. To
tell you the truth, I was also scared stiff. I kept thinking about
that film about the jockey you know, Bob Champion, who won
the Grand National. There was a scene when the poor man
looks at himself in the mirror and the chemo has made his hair
and eyebrows and eyelashes fall out. I thought, oh no, I couldn't
take that as well.

Many women, who just about cope with the profound nausea and
sickness, find the hair loss which may occur the final insult to an
already damaged body image, as can be seen in this harrowing
description by a 39-year-old woman who had undergone a mastectomy followed by radiotherapy and chemotherapy.

I've always been a fairly philosophical sort of person really, you
know. I tend to make the best of most things that happen, but
the chemotherapy beat me. I had just about coped with losing
my breast although I was rather worried about my partner's
reaction to it, but when my hair started to come out in handfuls
that finished me. I remember getting up one night after a
treatment session and being sick in the bathroom. I looked at
myself in the mirror and nearly fainted with shock. All my hair
had gone in one go. I just stood there naked looking at myself –
it was like a horror movie or a nightmare. I had one breast, and
no hair left anywhere. I broke down and cried for ages. I must
say that the only good thing that came out of it was that when
my hair grew back it was darker and curly. I rather liked that. I'd
never go through it again though.

Some of the modern chemotherapy drugs given to women with
breast cancer do not cause the total alopecia common in the past, but
nausea and/or vomiting remains a real problem for most patients.
Some women develop a powerful conditioned response to all aspects
of the treatment, so much so that the mere thought of going to the
hospital, seeing a needle, or the smell of a medi-swab are enough to
produce vomiting. This anticipatory vomiting and/or nausea can last
for many years, as can be seen in the following account of a 36-year-
old woman's ordeal.

I had to beg them to stop giving me the chemotherapy. I just couldn't face another course. After the second course I found that thinking about going there made me vomit – in fact it was almost as bad as when I was actually having the treatment. Even now (two years later) I start feeling sick when I pass by the hospital. I went there the other day to see a friend who had a baby, but I couldn't stay – that hospital smell brought it all back. I doubt that I could voluntarily put myself through chemotherapy again, even if I knew my life depended upon it.

Apart from the pronounced physical effects, there are many psychological side effects associated with chemotherapy. Maguire *et al.* (1980) studied the psychiatric morbidity of women who underwent mastectomy and CMF (Cyclophosphamide, Methotrexate and 5–Fluorouracil) or mastectomy alone. Significantly more of the women who received chemotherapy were rated as anxious and/or depressed. Those who had the most troublesome side effects were most likely to have severe anxiety and/or depression. An interesting and sad finding of this study was the revelation that many women had discussed neither their physical nor their psychological problems with their doctors. Some patients do not disclose the extent of their suffering to doctors for fear that 'life-saving' treatment will be stopped. There is a mistaken feeling that if treatment hurts then it must also be helping. Sadly, if patients fail to reveal their distress and discomfort, then their clinicians continue to underestimate the deleterious impact treatment may be having. Furthermore, they may not offer patients ameliorative treatment such as anti-emetics or psychological interventions such as relaxation therapy or desensitization for anticipatory nausea and vomiting. An example of this overly stoical attitude which resulted in a woman suffering in silence, for fear that treatment might be discontinued, can be seen in the following extract from an interview.

Interviewer: Just how bad did you get during the chemotherapy?
Patient: Rock bottom, about as far as it is possible to go.
Interviewer: Can you face describing what happened for me?
Patient: It got so bad that I started to shake days before I knew I was due to go. I was sick – I couldn't keep anything down.
Interviewer: Did you tell the doctors or nurses how bad you were feeling?
Patient: No, definitely not. I pretended everything was fine.

> I was quite determined to carry on and I thought
> that if I gave in and told them they might reduce the
> dose or stop giving it to me. I kept telling myself
> that if it was making me feel so awful then it must
> be doing its job.

Those patients who experience deep depression, anxiety, and other incapacitating physical side effects usually persevere with chemotherapy if they can believe that the net benefits are increased chances of survival. The research evidence to date from clinical trials reveals a statistical advantage to the pre-menopausal woman, but this does not necessarily translate into individual benefit. If a woman with breast cancer finds the gruelling side effects of treatment too intolerable, then encouragement to continue seems on balance rather difficult to justify. This is particularly true when palliation is the only realistic aim, as I shall discuss later in Chapter 5.

Once a woman has recovered from the immediate problems of coping with surgery, radiotherapy, and possibly chemotherapy, then various other psychosocial problems may surface. I have already discussed the high incidence of anxiety and depression post-treatment. Much of this psychiatric morbidity is due to the fear of having the dread disease, but other things may either contribute to, or result from, anxiety and depression. This includes such things as body image concerns, sexual dysfunction, and fear of recurrence.

Body image

> I know you'll think me a silly vain old thing, but quite honestly
> since the operation I just don't feel a woman anymore.

The quotation above comes from an interview with a 75-year-old spinster, who had never had a sexual partner. It demonstrates the necessity to regard all women with breast cancer as individuals. Far too often psychologically-damaging decisions are made based on assumptions that the elderly woman or the sexually inactive would not mind losing a breast, so a mastectomy is the operation performed. In one study sixty-two women with early breast cancer were given the option of choosing their surgical treatment. In the study, 19 (31 per cent) chose mastectomy and 43 (69 per cent) chose lumpectomy. Nearly all the women who chose mastectomy were 49 years or over, but 25 of the 43 women who chose lumpectomy (58 per cent) were also over the age of 50, and 13 of 21 (62 per cent) of women over the age of 60 opted for lumpectomy, demonstrating the fallacy that age is an appropriate criterion for determining treatment (Fallowfield *et al.* 1990).

Likewise, the assumption that the preservation of body image is the foremost preoccupation of younger sexually-active women is not borne out by research data. In our study of 269 women 12 per cent gave breast loss as their primary concern, 60 per cent gave fear of cancer as their worst thought and 19 per cent felt that both fear of disease and breast loss were equally distressing to contemplate.

One of the difficulties with much of the work cited earlier in this chapter is the problem of small sample size, inappropriate or biased sample composition, and the use of non-standardized measures for the assessment of body image. Nonetheless, the authors of these papers feel that the alteration to, and dissatisfaction with, body image following mastectomy means that lumpectomy should be the treatment of choice.

There is no logical reason for confidence in basing treatment decisions on such an argument. If an important visible part of one's body is amputated or mutilated then it stands to reason that body image will be affected. This in itself is obvious and tells us little about the impact that altered body image may have had on an individual woman's psychological or sexual functioning. It is possible for some women to feel dissatisfaction with body image but to cope well psychologically with breast loss. However, other women may have such a pronounced sense of body image that their psychological distress following mastectomy supercedes the contribution that having a life-threatening disease makes to psychological dysfunction. There are a few women who develop a pronounced self-consciousness following mastectomy; they feel sure that other people can tell that they have only one breast. Such women may become so distressed by this that they start wearing very baggy clothing to disguise their shape or become socially phobic and withdraw from interactions with other people.

> I am always worried that I'm not even. I tend to walk along with my arms folded to hide it. Whenever someone says 'Hello, how are you?' I always think that they are looking at my chest.

Simple reassurances that no one can tell seem to have little impact on psychosocial adjustment and these women may benefit from cognitive behaviour therapy which aims to promote more positive thinking, in particular, encouraging self-esteem (Maguire 1989). Some women cope well enough with self image when dressed, but experience considerable distress when unclothed.

Interviewer: Can you tell me how you felt about your appearance since your operation?

Patient: Mm, that depends – I think I look OK when I'm wearing my false one, don't you? I don't think anyone could tell.

Interviewer: And without your clothes?

Patient: That's rather different – I tend not to look at myself – it upsets me that I don't look like a woman any more.

Interviewer: What about when you're with your husband?

Patient: Oh, I don't let him see me, oh no, I couldn't. He'd be horrified. I always undress in the bathroom now.

The partners of women who have had a mastectomy may also profit from psychological help in adjusting to their partner's altered appearance. One early study reported by Jamison *et al.* (1978) revealed that 23 per cent of 41 women had not allowed their husbands to see them naked post-mastectomy.

Up to one-third of women feel very dissatisfied with their prosthesis; these dissatisfactions are usually due to worries that it will fall out or slip, making them look uneven. Some women complain that their prosthesis is too heavy, hot, or unwieldy. Such concerns may be understandable, but some women feel so disgusted by the sight and feel of their prosthetic breast, that occasionally body-image problems may manifest themselves in terms of hatred, revulsion, or phobic avoidance of the external prosthesis.

It is so revolting, it looks like a piece of filleted chicken breast. I can't bear to touch it, or to wash it. I'm still using the cotton wool temporary thing instead.

I think it's horrible – I get palpitations and go hot and cold whenever I touch it or think about it.

I hate it so much – last week I just felt so angry that they'd taken off my breast and given me that awful alien thing – I threw it across the room and cried.

The development of more successful implantation techniques and breast reconstruction may play a vital role in the rehabilitation of women who are devastated by breast loss. Dean *et al.* (1983) studied the psychosexual outcome in women randomized to either mastectomy and immediate reconstruction or mastectomy alone. At three months post-surgery significantly fewer (7 per cent) of the breast-implant group had signs of psychiatric morbidity than those women without an implant, of whom 36 per cent were experiencing probable psychiatric illness according to the General Health Questionnaire (GHQ). Unfortunately, sexual dysfunction was equally apparent in both groups. One important point to note about this study is that women were randomized. It would be interesting to study the psychosexual outcome in women permitted to choose their preferred option, that is either reconstruction or not. Most work to date suggests that provided women wish reconstruction for themselves and are not being pressurized by others to have one, and provided that they have realistic expectations of what can be achieved, then the outcome is very good.

Some researchers have reported that the dissatisfaction with body image may have less to do with fear of cancer and loss of a breast than was previously thought (Penman *et al.* 1987). In an interesting multi-centre study that compared self concept and social function in women being treated for a variety of non-cancer problems, such as cholecystectomy or benign breast disease, with that of women who underwent mastectomy for breast cancer, being overweight was the most important predictor of body-image dissatisfaction. Also correlated with a poorer body image were fewer social supports, concurrent medical problems, and a low internal score on locus of control.

Finally, not all women who undergo breast-conserving procedures are pleased with the cosmetic outcome. Some women in our study (13 per cent) felt that being told that they would only have to have the lump removed was misleading, as they expected to be left with symmetrical breasts (Fallowfield *et al.* 1987). Unfortunately, a wide local excision does not always produce a satisfactory result, especially if the woman is small breasted or has a lump very close to the nipple. Radiotherapy, unless skilfully done, can also produce most unpleasant skin thickening and discolouration. The following quotation shows that body image is not always preserved after breast-conserving surgery.

When he said they'd remove a little lump, I felt relieved. I mean no-one really wants to lose a breast do they? But when I look at what's left, I wonder if it was worth it. I mean, I'm still a freak aren't I? I don't like touching it and I'm scared to death it's going to come back again.

The wisest policy to pursue, based on current evidence, is to ask women about their own personal preferences if choice between treatments is technically feasible (see Chapter 7). Those women unable to make an informed decision due to ignorance about the appearance of the chest wall following mastectomy or the breast following the different sorts of excisions performed in breast-conserving surgery, may be helped by the provision of photographs. For those women with a pronounced sense of body image who have to undergo mastectomy for technical reasons, the option for breast reconstruction should *always* be mentioned and seen as an important part of treatment, not a trivial adjunct to therapy if resources permit. Finally, no woman should have her treatment determined on the basis of outmoded and incorrect assumptions that the elderly or single woman without a sexual partner would not be perturbed about breast loss, or that the young, sexually active woman always wants breast-conserving surgery.

Sexual dysfunction

In our culture powerful sexual stereotyping means that breasts have become symbolically linked to feelings of warmth, motherhood, affection, femininity, and sexuality. It is, therefore, no surprise to find that loss of a breast can create severe sexual dysfunction in the form of loss of self image, lowered self-esteem, a loss of perceived attractiveness, embarrassment or inhibition, and a loss of libido. Morris et al. (1977) reported a deterioration in sexual interest in 18 per cent of women studied by them three months post-mastectomy. At two years this figure had risen to 32 per cent, but so had the figure for women treated for benign breast disease. This report conflicts with that done by Maguire et al. (1978); they measured sexual activity prospectively in women treated for breast cancer by mastectomy or local excision for benign breast disease. Prior to surgery, 8 per cent of both groups had sexual problems. At four months post-treatment 40 per cent of the mastectomy group had problems in comparison to

12 per cent of the benign control group. At one year post-mastectomy 33 per cent were still experiencing moderate to severe difficulties whilst the control group remained the same with 12 per cent still reporting a loss of sexual interest and activity. As I have already mentioned in the previous sections, it is naive to presume that breast loss alone is the cause of psychological problems; likewise sexual dysfunction may be due to factors other than mastectomy for significant numbers of women.

Two more recent studies measured the level of sexual interest using a self-report item from the Rotterdam Symptom Checklist (RSCL) in women who underwent either a mastectomy or breast-sparing surgery for early breast cancer (Fallowfield et al. 1986; Fallowfield et al. 1990). In both studies the sexual interest of previously sexually-active women had declined in well over one quarter of the respondents, irrespective of their surgical treatment. This loss of libido in women who have not suffered breast loss appears to be a counterintuitive finding and is therefore worthy of more research work. Possible hypotheses are that the diagnosis of cancer and/or radiotherapy cause depression which produces a loss of libido.

The impact of adjuvant therapy on sexuality was demonstrated by Penman et al. (1987). They found that women who had adjuvant radiotherapy and/or chemotherapy expressed more concern about physical affection, sexual relationships, and feelings of femininity or sexual attractiveness than women treated by mastectomy alone. Indeed, the mastectomy alone group showed no significant differences on any of these issues from women being treated for non-cancer problems. Likewise Silberfarb et al. (1980) reported that radiotherapy and/or chemotherapy lessened sexual desire in women being treated for breast cancer. Some women also complain that they lose a considerable amount of sensation in the affected breast following radiotherapy or that their partners seem reluctant to touch the breast. The following quotation is from an interview with a 39-year-old woman for whom body image was an important consideration when choosing her surgical treatment. She had a very bad skin reaction during radiotherapy.

I've gone right off sex since this business started. The reason I wouldn't let them take it off [her breast] was because my old man is very keen on breasts, if you know what I mean. But then

> I had all this burning and itching during the radium and my skin is still awful. I can't stand anything tight, clothes and that, and if he comes near me or touches it well I just hit the roof. I'm conscious of my breast all the time – it's really ruined our sex life.

If breasts were an important source of sexual stimulation prior to surgery then couples may need to find other means of enhancing desire and enjoyment of love-making.

One area worth exploring with couples who are experiencing sexual difficulties following treatment for breast cancer concerns their beliefs about causal factors in the disease. Fear of contagion is much more widespread than most health carers imagine, as are worries that sexual activity will promote the likelihood of recurrence and that cancer is a punishment for past sexual indiscretions. Some partners of cancer patients worry that they will be exposed to radiation if they touch their wife's breast while she is undergoing radiotherapy (Schover and Jensen 1988).

The psychological impact of a diagnosis of cancer and treatment may make a woman so overwhelmingly preoccupied with thoughts of survival, anger about the unfairness of becoming a victim, uncertainty about the future, and so forth that sexual desire is rather low down on the list of priorities, as the following extract from an interview demonstrates.

Interviewer: Has all this affected your sexual relationship with your husband at all?

Patient: Sex – you must be joking – that's the last thing I can think about. I'm so tired and so on edge it wouldn't be worth him even touching me. I've got too much to worry about to be bothered with sex.

Some authors have stated that even good, stable marriages are placed under considerable strain by mastectomy (Wabrek and Wabrek 1976). Other writers, such as Maguire (1985), have high-lighted the importance that spouses play in the psychosexual rehabilitation of women with breast cancer. Those men who were able to provide positive support in the form of reaffirmation of love and affection and who prevented their wives from concealing their scars and/or encouraged social and sexual contact, greatly assisted the recovery of their partners.

For some couples the trauma of breast cancer actually brings them closer together, as can be seen in this extract.

You hear so much these days about men going off with younger women. I must admit I didn't really think about the cancer and losing my life. I was more worried about losing my husband when he saw what I looked like. He's never been much good at illness and things. It's funny though, you know, he was really great and told me that it wasn't breasts he'd married, but me, and he'd rather have me with one breast, one arm, one eye, one leg, than not at all. If anything, the physical side of things – you know, sex and that – is better than it's been for years.

Not all men react in this way and some find that they too lose sexual desire for their wives. It is unclear whether this is due to physical revulsion and finding their partners less sexually attractive (especially following mastectomy and during chemotherapy), or due to depression and anxiety at the thought that their partner has a life-threatening disease. Following an interview that I had with a woman in her own home, her husband accompanied me to the garden gate and asked who was available to help him. He claimed to still love his wife, but felt so distressed by her changed appearance and her changed mood that he could not see how their relationship could survive. It seems clear that most stable relationships can weather the trauma, but that fragile relationships are easily broken by the stress and strain of breast cancer treatment.

Fear of recurrence

Fear of recurrence seems a pre-eminent worry for most women, especially during the first few years following diagnosis and treatment. According to Ray and Baum (1985), the woman with breast cancer 'has to come to terms not so much with death as with the unpredictability of the future and with the ambiguity of her current status. She is neither clearly ill nor clearly healthy; her status is one of "at risk" (Baric 1969). A feature of this "at risk" role is that even the most optimistic patient may be alert for symptoms that could mean that the disease has recurred.' This worry can be identified very clearly in the following quotations.

I'm just frightened now in case I find another lump. It's preying on my mind all the time that there's been one and I might get another one, you know.

Some women who experience this crippling anxiety that the cancer will return, may exhibit hypervigilant monitoring of the body for signs of the dreaded recurrence. Every bodily ache or pain is interpreted as cancer.

Do you know, if I get a pain in my stomach now it's got to be cancer; if I've got a pain in my back I'm going to get lung cancer; get a bad head, I'm getting a tumour on the brain. I just can't get it out of my head.

Some women with breast cancer, especially those who have had breast-conserving therapy, develop obsessional checking of their breasts. In one study Fallowfield *et al.* (1987) reported that 10 per cent of their sample of women admitted to at least daily self-examination. This is an important observation when one considers how few women in this country ever practise breast self-examination (see Chapter 2).

I just cannot keep my hand off [my breast]. It's something that I've never ever done. I spend hours just lying there feeling, and when I touch I feel as if I've got lumps all over.

The doctor faces a dilemma when trying to help the obsessionally anxious woman who fears recurrence. Simple reassurances and repeated mammograms or bone scans do little to allay the overly anxious. The help of an experienced counsellor or psychologist who can offer relaxation therapy and/or desensitization is probably necessary for those women with severe obsessions. (A useful guide to coping with breast cancer which includes clear instructions for patients wanting to practise relaxation techniques can be found in Tarrier, 1987.)

The transition from a fit, active, and happy woman to a person with breast cancer and all that the diagnosis and treatment entails can be very quick and may contribute to some of the adjustment difficulties experienced. An account of this rapid transition can be seen in the following passage taken from an interview with a 45-year-old successful business woman. Her breast cancer had been found after a routine examination at a Well-Woman clinic revealed a small lump. She had a mastectomy within a week, followed by a course of radiotherapy. Twelve months later she was still not back at work and felt very depressed and anxious.

> Looking back over this past year is like a bad dream. One minute I was a successful business woman running my own company. The future looked very bright. I had 42 people working for me and I really felt that I was, well that I was *living*. I'd felt so healthy – I often got tired of course, if we'd had a particularly busy stretch. I suppose that was the most difficult thing to accept. I felt so well and yet the cancer had been there for some time. I felt as though my body had let me down and I couldn't trust it any more. I know why you were asking me if I checked my other breast for lumps. The truth is I'm doing it all the time, as I'm terrified that it's going to come back, but then I get upset and panicky – I mean I didn't find the first one did I? I don't see myself as a cured person. I feel irretrievably changed now – not just because I'm physically different without a breast, but I'm mentally different. I went overnight from a confident, articulate person to someone who can't even answer the telephone. I'm constantly scared – the sheer joy of living has gone out of me.

Some women say that they never feel really sure that their cancer has been cured – at best it has been held in check. In the words of one such woman, '... one of the things is, I don't know whether to say, you know, to myself, well you've *had* cancer... or whether one should say you've *got* cancer, you are still a cancer patient.'

Clearly the diagnosis and treatment of breast cancer changes women's lives, but not always in a detrimental way. I shall end this chapter with a happier, more optimistic quotation from a 34-year-old woman with breast cancer who had two young children.

> I can honestly say that the cancer has made me a better, more tolerant person. I used to get upset and irritable about the most stupid things. Having breast cancer has put everything in perspective. I treasure each minute of life. Who wants the shiniest kitchen floor when you could be out on the Downs walking instead, or playing with the children? I took so many things for granted before this happened and wasted so much time on things that don't matter. Having breast cancer has changed all that – I value the smallest thing – I'm grateful in a way, although it's a rather drastic way in which to suddenly see the light!

Chapter five

Psychological reactions to recurrence and advanced disease

Recurrence: feelings on finding another breast lump

I just went cold – I knew instantly what it was. I suppose in my heart of hearts I'd always expected it to come back, in spite of what they'd told me. I didn't really cry or anything. I just made an appointment to see my GP and wondered what I should tell the family.

One might predict that the emotional impact of recurrent breast cancer would be devastating. All the hopes and confidence that treatment had been successful, together with long-term plans for the woman's future, are shattered and need rethinking. Confidence, adaptation, and adjustment usually increase over time and the longer the interval that has elapsed since initial diagnosis, the more hopeful and optimistic women become that they have been cured. All the emotional distress described earlier, when women first find a breast lump or hear their diagnosis, may resurface when they realize that the cancer has returned, but is there any evidence that recurrence, which may shatter optimism about cure, is more disturbing than the initial diagnosis? There is surprisingly little research in this particular area in contrast to the voluminous work about early stage disease. Some writers have suggested that recurrence provokes more emotional distress than that found in newly-diagnosed cancer patients (Holland 1977), although this has rarely been formally tested. Weisman and Worden (1986) reported data from a study of 102 mixed cancer patients including women with breast cancer. They found that 30 per cent of patients thought recurrence less traumatic than the original diagnosis.

We have found in our own work that the reactions of women who discover that they have yet another lump vary enormously. Some women claim a strange sense of relief in that they had always felt anxious that the cancer would return and therefore the diagnosis of recurrence ends the uncertainty. This reaction may be similar to that experienced by women awaiting diagnosis at the beginning of their disease who, after finding the initial lump, experience crippling anxiety that they have cancer and subsequent relief when the diagnosis has been confirmed (see Chapter 3). Other women treat the news of recurrence with such equanimity that one might suppose that they have mentally rehearsed the scenario sufficient times for the shock to be somewhat attenuated. These women tend to adopt a practical and philosophical approach. They may worry more about the distress that the news about recurrence will have on their families than about the further treatment that they themselves must confront again. The quotation at the beginning of this chapter is typical of women who react with stoicism or an attitude of preparedness.

This type of reaction fits with the models of coping in cancer described by Lloyd (1979) and Rosch (1981), both of whom suggest that cancer patients are chronically stressed by the ever-present threat of recurrence (The Sword-of-Damocles syndrome) and are not surprised therefore when the cancer actually does recur. Weisman and Worden (1986) reported a correlation between the degree of emotional distress experienced by women at the time of their recurrence and the degree of expectation of recurrence. Most women who are surprised by the return of their cancer are extremely distressed, fearful, and some are angry. Frequently expressed feelings include 'Why me?', 'What have I done, or not done?' Other women may demonstrate very hostile reactions to the rest of the 'well' world and engage in comparisons of their own behaviour or goodness relative to the evil behaviour of others who either do not have cancer or appear to have been cured of their disease. The following quotation displays this reaction most vividly.

> Oh I cried and cried and thought, it isn't fair after all I've been through already. It isn't, is it? What have I done to deserve all this? I don't believe in God, but I've led what you'd call a Christian life, unlike some people I know. Why should I suffer even more?

Such attitudes relate back to the issues of causal factors in cancer discussed earlier in Chapter 2 where cancer could be viewed by some as 'punishment' for past misdemeanours. From a counselling point of view, women with pronounced 'just world' expectations can be very hard to help and this area will be discussed further in Chapter 6.

One potential problem for those women who have had breast-conserving procedures is that of assuming guilt or feeling responsible for the recurrence. A good example can be seen in the comments that follow, which were made by a 51-year-old woman who had just learned that she had to undergo a mastectomy for locally-recurring breast cancer.

> I'm so upset and it's stupid of me really – I should have had the mastectomy in the first place. Mr H. told me that was what he'd recommended, but I just insisted – they weren't going to take my breast – but now it's back – I suppose you could say it's my fault for being vain.

Fortunately the surgeon can still reassure women with local recurrence that further effective treatment is available and that there is no reason to suppose that the return of the cancer is necessarily anything to do with her behaviour, either in the past or the present. However, there are some data emerging which suggest that recurrent disease may be provoked by emotional distress following noxious life events. Ramirez and her colleagues (1989) studied 100 women with breast cancer, 50 of whom had developed recurrence and 50 matched controls, who were disease-free. They found that severely-threatening life events and difficulties, such as bereavement or family breakdown, were significantly associated with first recurrence of breast cancer. The authors themselves caution that the study needs to be confirmed using a prospective design with a larger population, but their report attracted widespread publicity. Following a newspaper article about the Ramirez study a woman in one of our studies telephoned to find out more; she felt that her recently diagnosed recurrence could have been due to the stress caused by her husband leaving her a few months previously.

Coping with further treatment

If a woman has a local recurrence and no evidence of metastatic spread then there are still some further treatments that can promote a realistic prospect of survival. Those women who originally had a breast-conserving operation may have a mastectomy and others may be given radiotherapy and/or hormonal or cytotoxic chemotherapy (see Chapter 1). Some women who require a mastectomy for locally-recurring disease are angry and feel that the primary therapy must have compromised their survival chances. Below is a typical expression of the anger and concern felt by a 49-year-old woman who had just been told by her GP that the lump in her breast was probably recurrent disease:

> I thought, oh no, not again. I phoned up straight away and demanded to see Mr H. I was more angry than scared. I'd asked him you see if it was safer to have a mastectomy, but he said it made no difference. Now I've ended up having to have another operation and more time off work.

The prospect of further treatment worries certain women more than their fear of recurrent cancer.

> I suppose that you always have this nagging doubt that you're really living on borrowed time, so it wasn't exactly a surprise – I wasn't ever that sure that they'd cured me. Though I was prepared for the cancer to come back sometime, I hadn't really thought what they'd – what the next treatment might be. I knew they wouldn't try the radium again, so it had to be either chemotherapy or a mastectomy. I was very worried about that – I knew I wouldn't cope very well.

Some patients feel that coping with treatment is much tougher the second time around as they do not have the same degree of optimism about their future as the following two quotations show.

> I knew I needed the radiotherapy, but I was totally against the chemotherapy because I couldn't see the value in making myself ill. You know you always think in terms of you will be the one who gets away – and obviously now, I know that clearly in my case that was not true and I must think more seriously about it.

> I didn't respond very well after the operation this time. Everyone was amazed at how quickly I recovered after the first operation – I was up and about the next day joking about and handing out the teas on the ward. I felt so relieved and happy that it was all over. I was convinced that everything was going to work out fine. This second lump in the other breast was a real

blow – I'm not so sure that I'm going to be one of the lucky ones after all. The operation hurt more, I got a wound infection around the scar you know, and I still can't move my arm on that side properly, it's all so swollen. I'm a bit nervous about the future now.

I have already mentioned the dearth of data from formal assessments comparing psychological distress at first diagnosis with that at recurrence. Therefore my comments are based on mainly anecdotal observations from interviews with patients. These discussions convey an impression of distress, concern about further treatment, and renewed worries about long-term survival. However, the majority of women do appear prepared for the cancer to return and provided that the support systems marshalled together in the earlier stages of their breast cancer remain intact, then most seem to cope fairly well.

Advanced breast cancer

The treatment of patients with advanced breast cancer has provoked considerable controversy. Sadly, any woman with advanced metastatic disease is condemned to die within a few months. Thus, supportive therapy aimed at producing palliation of symptoms is the only realistic therapy for a clinician to offer. Too often, particularly in the USA, active therapy involving unpleasantly toxic chemotherapy is given, despite there being little evidence to date of any real survival benefit to the patient. In the treatment of advanced breast disease, the only criterion of benefit should be quality of life (Fallowfield and Baum 1989).

Unfortunately, some of the statistically significant signs of apparent response to chemotherapy treatment which might excite the clinician may be of little significance to the patient. A balance has to be struck between providing a modest extension to life at the cost of intolerable side effects and 'cytotoxic therapies that could produce tumour shrinkage and some prolongation of life might not be considered as beneficial to the patient if those precious extra months are spent with the miseries of alopecia, nausea, vomiting, and mouth soreness' (Clark and Fallowfield 1986). There are women for whom *any* chance of gaining an extension of life is deemed worth the toxicity and provided that they have been given an honest description of the likely benefits and side effects, it seems unfair to deny them treatment. The following two quotations show very different reactions experienced by two women contemplating further treatment with chemotherapy for advanced disease. The first is from an interview with a 32-year-old woman with two young children, who felt prepared to embark on any treatment which might have increased her survival chances: 'Well I just said to him, I don't care how slim the chances are or what the side-effects might be – I'll try anything.'

Responses such as these are fairly common, but the doctor should ensure that the patient really has been given an unbiased description of the true benefits likely to accrue.

The second quotation is from a woman who felt quite certain that she wanted only that treatment likely to ease any pain. She hated the thought of any more active therapy or time spent in hospital.

> He was very honest and very kind at the same time. I said that
> I'd talk it over with the family, but I knew really that I wasn't
> going to have any more of that chemotherapy. They said that
> some radiotherapy for my spine would help the pain, so I agreed
> to that, but I hate being sick and just the thought of the
> chemotherapy last time made me ill. I'm alright now I've got
> used to the idea that my time is nearly up. I want to be at home,
> not in hospital really ill with drips and things.

Occasionally some altruistic women are prepared to volunteer for Phase I and II clinical trials of new therapies. They may gain considerable psychological benefit from the knowledge that results of such work may help others.

> I don't want to die for nothing. I'll try anything if it will help
> them [doctors] to find a cure. My daughters or granddaughters
> might get it – I'd like to think I'd helped.

However, active therapy in advanced breast cancer should only be offered as part of a properly conducted clinical trial following informed consent. Extending the implicit promise to patients that participating in such research may be of significant individual benefit to them is not ethical.

A woman with metastatic breast cancer still has need of good practical medical care, even though this has no curative intent. The physical support required at this time concerns primarily the control of pain affecting all the sites of metastatic spread. Breast cancer tends to metastasize to the brain, lung, and/or bone. It is the latter site, that of bone, which usually produces the most intractable pain and palliative radiotherapy can often bring substantial relief. Another distressing physical symptom of advanced disease is hypercalcaemia which can produce mood disorders and cognitive changes. These confusional states may require psychiatric intervention and drugs such as Haloperidol have been shown to help (Massie *et al.* 1983).

Psychological morbidity

In contrast to the large volume of research reporting psychological morbidity in early breast cancer, there has been surprisingly little work looking at the specific problems of those with advanced disease. Most studies done on patients suffering from advanced cancer at a variety of different sites, report that between 25–50 per cent of patients are depressed and/or anxious at any one time. Depression seems to dominate; for example, Plumb and Holland (1977) studied ninety-seven patients with advanced cancer and found 23 per cent to be either moderately or severely depressed. In a later series, Plumb and Holland (1981) reported clinically-significant depression in 20–30 per cent of patients admitted for treatment of advanced cancer.

Bukberg and colleagues (1984) have suggested that depression, to some extent, depends on the degree of physical disability in that patients who are physically exhausted become emotionally exhausted as well. Using the Karnofsky Performance Index, Bukberg *et al.* found that of those patients with very low scores (40 or less) 77 per cent had symptoms of major depressive illness, whereas amongst those patients with scores of 60 or more indicating good physical performance, only 23 per cent had symptoms consistent with a major depression.

The studies mentioned so far have been on mixed cancer patients. Hopwood (1984) looked at psychiatric morbidity in twenty-six women with metastatic breast cancer admitted for chemotherapy before and two to three months after their cytotoxic therapy. She found 35 per cent of women to be anxious or depressed, with reaction depression the most common psychological problem. The majority of the anxious and depressed women responded well to anxiolytic or anti-depressant therapy, demonstrating once more the need to make psychiatric assessment and then appropriate intervention part of the routine clinical management.

Some of the depressive illness found in patients with advanced cancer may be due to organic brain syndromes, for example cerebral metastases or metabolic disturbances caused by liver failure or hypercalcaemia. Establishing the primary underlying problem causing the depression is very important; anti-depressant therapy, for example, is unlikely to help a patient with an organic brain syndrome find relief from depression, whereas a short course of radiotherapy might be effective. There are other reasons for depression in advanced disease, including such things as fear of death, worrying about becoming a burden to the family, and considerable distress at the prospect of no longer being able to care for relatives. This major role-loss for a woman with breast cancer may be particularly disturbing if she has children or others dependent upon her, as the following quotations from two women with terminal breast cancer reveal. The first patient was married with two children and beginning to doubt the wisdom of her decision to die at home.

> The worst thing of all isn't that I know I'm dying, it's worrying about the children. R. [her husband] has never done much for them and now he's got to do everything for me, for himself and for them. It makes me feel a complete failure to them all. I'm beginning to think they'd be better off with me in hospital instead of here where I'm an extra burden.

The second patient was a 43-year-old single woman who still lived with her elderly, rather frail, mother.

> I've not been doing at all well since you last saw me – I look pretty awful don't I? I'm so depressed. My poor old Mum shouldn't be having to cope with this – she should be able to put her feet up and have me looking after her, not the other way round. I keep wondering what will happen to her when I'm gone. Sometimes I think I've been nothing but trouble for her ever since I was born.

Although a significant minority of women with advanced disease suffer anxiety and depression, some authors have suggested that their problems are not as severe as that found following the discovery of recurrent cancer. Silberfarb *et al.* (1980) compared psychiatric morbidity of three groups of breast cancer patients at different stages of disease. They reported a greater frequency of depression, anxiety, and suicidal ideation amongst those women recently found to have a recurrence than in those terminally ill.

Effect on relatives

The news that a woman has recurrence or has advanced disease may be deeply stressful for her relatives.

Husband: I'm finding it very hard to think straight – to know what to do or say to her. I can't stop work as we obviously need the money, yet I'm aware when I'm at work that she is alone at home and that she won't be here much longer. I suppose that I don't really want to believe that this is happening. I can't imagine life without her yet, she isn't the same person any more – she looks so different and she is so different. Oh God, it's like she's dead already.

Interviewer: I'm sorry you're so upset – perhaps, it would help to talk about this a little more? It sounds to me as though you are really telling me that you are continuing to work because it helps you avoid the reality of what's happening to your wife?

Husband: Yes – that's it – sometimes when I'm busy I can forget for a bit, but then it all comes back and I get this awful pit in my stomach. I feel guilty and useless. I loved her so much you see, she was so, so pretty and full of life – I can't bear to see her as she is – I don't want her to die, but I don't think I can take much more of seeing her like this. I'm scared about her dying – I don't know what I'll do.

Interviewer: Have you both been able to talk about any of this with each other?

Husband: God – no! You must be joking – that would be like admitting it wouldn't it. She mustn't give up hope.

This extract from a lengthy interview with a 40-year-old man whose wife had advanced breast cancer, provides a poignant example of some of the dilemmas and stresses that confront the partners of terminally-ill patients. This man was finding it very hard to face the reality of what was happening. His primary means of coping, that of avoidance, was not really working and he was consumed with guilt about ambivalent feelings. On the one hand he could not bear the thought of his wife's death, yet he could not cope with watching her dying. He wished for her release from suffering and his own release from witnessing the suffering, yet the price of this release was her death which he found unacceptable. Such reactions are not uncommon and demonstrate the need for professional counselling support to be made available for the spouses and partners of women dying from breast cancer.

In a study reported by Gotay (1984) of women with advanced breast cancer and their partners, talking about it to others was the most useful coping strategy.

Another important practical issue raised by the extract from the interview is that of facilitating communication between the dying woman and her partner. Some couples find it extremely difficult to discuss what is happening with each other. They might both be attempting to protect each other, but usually end up feeling distant and unsupported at a time when they need each other most. It is very sad to witness, 'Couples, instead of drawing closer together, wither in each other's arms' (Goldie 1982).

Gotay's study found that men were much more disturbed by the thought of their partner's imminent death than the women themselves were. She reported that 'fear of death per se is not as dominant a problem for patients as it is for the people around them'.

The doctor/patient relationship

When advanced disease has been established, the psychological support required by both patients and their families is substantial and every bit as important as the necessity for good symptom control.

Patients and their families require an honest appraisal of their condition – which should include reassurance that their pain will be effectively controlled. Extending unrealistic expectations of response to more active therapy or colluding with relatives in maintaining a myth that cure is still possible rather than preparing the patient for death, may bring short-term comfort to everyone but increases distress when things obviously start to go wrong. A patient who has been deceived about her prognosis by doctors and nurses (albeit for mistaken, kindly, and protective motives) will not believe their reassurances that she will suffer no loss of dignity, no pain, or that she will not be left to die alone.

Some doctors insist that patients should not be told the truth about their advanced disease as this knowledge leaves the sufferers without hope that anything more can be done for them. This is a misinterpretation of what constitutes total care for a patient with breast cancer; symptom control in advanced disease *is* care, just as active therapy was care at the beginning of the woman's treatment. In the words of Holland and Rowland (1989); 'there is never a time that *nothing* can be done; comfort care in the face of advancing illness is an integral part of continuity of care'.

The appeal of alternative and unorthodox therapies

Patients who feel that nothing more *will be* done for them, rather than nothing more honestly *can be* done in terms of active therapy, may be easy prey for the pedlars of quack cures or remedies. Many of the patients who took part in a study of the drug Laetrile, for example, did so because they felt that 'medicine had failed them' (Redding *et al.* 1981). Other patients, often encouraged by friends and relatives, may seek out unorthodox alternative practitioners. I wish to make a firm distinction between blatant quackery and some of the other alternative therapies. The former category consists of charlatans and opportunists of the most unpleasant kind; they are offering 'cures' which are at best innocuous and at worst downright dangerous, for the sole purpose of extracting money out of desperate and gullible people. The quacks produce fraudulent, anecdotal evidence to support their claims for miracle cures and contribute nothing to the long-term physical or psychological well-being of their victims.

Other unorthodox alternative practitioners tend to have rather different motives. Most of these people have as their primary aim that of helping patients with cancer, and genuinely believe in the efficacy of their treatments. Unfortunately, they do not apply scientific method when evaluating their methods and rely almost entirely on corroborative data in the form of anecdotal case reports or testimonies. Michael Baum, one of the founder members of Healthwatch, the Campaign Against Fraud in Medicine, has written some vigorous rebuttals of the use of alternative remedies in breast cancer. As professor of surgery at a leading London teaching hospital, with a special interest in the proper scientific evaluation of treatments for breast cancer, he became increasingly concerned at the lack of intellectual honesty being displayed by many of the alternative cancer therapists. He, after all, often saw the results of homoeopathic remedies, naturopathy and aromatherapy in patients sent to him with advanced metastatic disease. Baum (1989) claims that one of the reasons that patients seek out alternative therapies is borne out of a sense of frustration that medical innovation and discovery appears to have slowed down as far as chronic diseases such as breast cancer are concerned. He claims that as the public have 'come to expect medical breakthroughs on demand in every decade and, with this frustration, we witness the emergence and self-confidence of the irrational schools of medicine, disguised as alternative or "holistic" medicine'.

Whilst evidence for the efficacy of alternative therapies is lacking, some clearly have much to offer certain patients in terms of maintaining hope and a sense of control. Women at all stages of breast cancer may be attracted to alternative therapies, some of which have a gentler image than the unpleasant conventional treatments such as radiotherapy or chemotherapy. Most women with breast cancer experience, at some time during the course of their disease, a profound sense of helplessness, provoked by the knowledge that their body harbours a tumour over which they have no control. They worry about the fact that cancer cells may spread throughout their body and that doctors can give no copper-bottomed guarantee that conventional therapy has eradicated the disease. Treatments are unpleasant and require high technological equipment which is frightening and increases the sense of dependency and loss of control. Finally, the absence of a proper understanding of breast cancer biology provides few clues as to its cause and therefore few clues as to what an individual woman can do to prevent its recurrence. Against such a backdrop it is hardly surprising that patients seek out alternative or unorthodox remedies. Although this can happen at any stage of the disease, it is often tried in a last ditch attempt to fight off cancer when all else appears to have failed or when a woman cannot face the thought of conventional therapy again.

When he said, 'I'm afraid it's cancer again', I thought, 'Oh no, I'm just not going through any more of that chemotherapy or radiotherapy business again.' It didn't cure me last time did it? So I wasn't going to put myself through that hell again. I found an article in a woman's magazine about diet and mind over matter and thought that it was likely to be worth a chance.

One appeal of unorthodox treatments is that they help maintain hope and promote a sense of self-sufficiency. The patient may feel in control of her body again and the more complex the diet or mental imaging demanded, the more this feeling of having regained some power or mastery over the disease is fostered. Another important attraction of unorthodox therapy is that it clearly meets many of the unmet emotional needs of women with breast cancer; needs that many traditional clinicians are either unwilling to address or inept at fulfilling. If women received more emotional support from their clinicians and other health-care professionals, then their desire to seek out help from the alternative practitioners would probably be less. However, to quote Michael Baum (1986) again: 'Doctors obviously need to try harder, but surely it is incredibly naive to believe that bedside manner alone is a sufficient alternative to truly effective cancer therapy.'

There is not room in this book for a comprehensive review of all the quack cures, folk and quasi-medical remedies that have been advocated at one time or another for cancer patients. The American Cancer Society (1983) catalogued at least 70 different unproven methods which included a variety of diets, drugs, and pseudo-psychological techniques. Some of these methods demand that their own diagnostic and testing materials or paraphernalia are used. Needless to say, this equipment is usually extremely expensive and the scientific rationale for its use or empirical evidence for its efficacy is lacking. To a lay population both the alternative and quack remedies do appear to have some logical appeal. Most are based on the notion that cancer is caused by some underlying systemic disorder, dysfunction, or toxicity requiring 'detoxification'; hence the need for such seemingly bizarre things as coffee enemas and 'pure' foods. Vegan-type diets are very popular; their appeal stems from the fact that cancer cells divide and multiply more rapidly than normal cells and as all cells require protein, those patients who avoid protein will starve the cancer cells. Unfortunately, the non-cancerous cells suffer as well. Consequently the patients, physically compromised by disease, can be weakened further by an inadequate diet. Interested readers should try the excellent article by Cassileth (1986) who surveyed alternative cancer cures promoted over the past 150 years. The observations of Lerner (1985) who visited thirty different alternative cancer centres is also highly recommended.

Most of the more respectable alternative treatment centres combine diet with megavitamins and some form of psychological approach such as the Simonton model (Simonton *et al.* 1980) used at the Bristol Cancer Help Centre. These psychological and spiritual approaches fit in with the stress hypothesis for cancer discussed in Chapter 2, which is popular amongst lay people and some researchers.

My view of many of these programmes, based on the experiences of patients who have been through them, are very mixed. Some individuals undoubtedly gain enormous benefit from the spiritual support and feeling that they are in control of their own bodies again. Others crumple under the physical and emotional strain of following the diet and assuming responsibility for the success or failures of treatment. There are few sadder sights than an emaciated, seriously-ill woman, with orange-tinted skin due to the vast quantities of carrot juice that her diet demands she drinks, desperately trying to fight the cancer and feeling overwhelmingly guilty about the fact that she is losing the battle because she hasn't 'fought' hard enough. The following example is taken from an interview with a young woman dying from advanced breast cancer. She was 34 years old, married with two young children and had undergone a mastectomy followed by chemotherapy 18 months previously. When she was diagnosed as having metastatic breast cancer, her husband and friends all encouraged her to go to the Bristol Cancer Care Centre. There she was given a special diet and taught their programme of imaging cancer cells being attacked and her body fighting back. She had been following the 'vegetarian' diet for three months and found the carrot juice unpalatable and the need to maintain a 'fighting spirit' exhausting. She felt consumed by guilt about the fact that she was obviously going to die shortly and wanted to give up the programme. The counsellor encouraged her to discuss this with her caring and supportive husband.

I just cracked and told H. [her husband] that I couldn't do it any more. He said it was all right and went out and bought some fillet steak. He'd hated the diet too, but thought that I'd have been upset and realise I was dying if he'd suggested we stopped. Somehow we seem closer and happier than we've ever been now we've stopped pretending what's going to happen to me. I've got more time to think about all the good things that have happened to us instead of concentrating on cancer cells all the time. I've been a very lucky person with the job I had, the husband I had and the children. It would have been nice to be around for grandchildren, but really I've known a lot of love in my life. Not everyone has that, do they?

(Quoted from Fallowfield 1990)

Conclusion

The clinical course of breast cancer is uncertain and most women harbour fears that the disease may return. For those with good social support and reassuring medical support these fears may abate with time, but some patients may develop such an obsessional, anxious preoccupation with the fear of recurrence that skilled psychological intervention may be necessary. The reactions of women to obvious disease progression is usually sadness and sometimes despair. Lack of appropriate care and support at this time may add to the burden and make women easy prey for the pedlars of quack cures and remedies. Some alternative therapies may contribute to a woman's sense of well-being and quality of life by giving them a sense of mastery and control. However, these approaches can produce some negative effects; in particular, no woman dying from breast cancer should have to endure the added burden of responsibility for disease progression.

Chapter six

Psychological interventions

The previous chapters in this book have described the myriad of emotional, social, and physical difficulties experienced by women at different stages of their disease. It should be obvious that any therapeutic approach that dismisses or ignores the substantial impact that psychological factors have on good outcome and long term adjustment is both poor medicine and poor science. The breast-care specialist nurse or oncology counsellor plays a vital role in the rehabilitation of women with breast cancer and a clear need exists for counselling support of the patient and her family, especially during terminal illness. The clinical psychologist may also help those women who develop such things as phobic reactions to their prosthesis, social and sexual avoidance, and obsessional checking of their bodies for signs of disease recurrence. Those women unfortunate enough to experience classically conditioned responses to chemotherapy, especially the distressing anticipatory nausea and vomiting, may find relief following desensitization and/or relaxation and stress management training. Finally, the liaison psychiatrist may supplement these interventions with psychotherapy and pharmacological treatment in the form of anxiolytics or anti-depressants for those patients with serious unremitting anxiety and/or depression.

In this chapter I shall discuss some of the specific counselling needs of women at different stages of breast cancer; I shall look briefly at some of the evidence for the efficacy of counselling and other interventions and provide illustrative examples of counselling from the case histories of women with breast cancer, whom I have myself counselled or interviewed about their counselling experiences.

Table 6.1 Strategies used in counselling women with breast cancer

1	*Directive*: The counsellor acts prescriptively, directing the behaviour of the woman wanting help
2	*Informative*: Providing information, giving help with decision-making, and helping understanding
3	*Confrontational*: Challenging unhelpful thinking or coping strategies that are hindering the patient coming to terms with the problem and providing feedback to enable patients to adapt and recognize negative thinking themselves
4	*Cathartic*: Permitting patients to express and release hidden thoughts, fears, and guilts in a safe non-judgemental setting, so encouraging better self-understanding
5	*Catalytic*: Being reflective and encouraging women to establish their own achievable goals, thus promoting a sense of control
6	*Supportive*: Providing the woman, and her family if necessary, with genuine, non-judgemental, empathetic support

Counselling needs at different stages

The primary aim in counselling patients with breast cancer is to help women find their own means of coping with the emotional stresses of having a life-threatening illness. By *coping* I refer to the helpful definition of Lazarus and Folkman (1984) which is 'constantly changing cognitive and behavioural efforts to manage specific external and/or internal demands that are appraised as taxing or exceeding the resources of the person'. The outcome of good coping in this sense means successfully adapting to the difficult and changing physical and emotional demands placed on a woman with breast cancer. I have already shown how the reactions of individuals may fluctuate between euphoria and despair, supreme optimism of cure and excessive pessimism about the outcome of treatment. At different times women may be beset and bemused by feelings of anger, guilt, fear, uncertainty, depression, and confusion about what to do and what the future holds. Effective counselling and psychotherapy should permit appropriate expression and ventilation of these negative emotions and then help the woman develop some more positive means of dealing with them by, for example, restructuring, channelling, or changing the way in which they perceive their current situation and perceive their future. In common with counselling in any setting, most counselling of women with breast cancer contains essentially the six primary approaches or strategies summarized in Table 6.1 (see also Fallowfield 1988).

The eclectic, well-trained counsellor uses all these forms of approach, or elements of them, at different times with different patients, as can be seen in the following examples.

Counselling needs at diagnosis

Directive and informative, cathartic and supportive counselling approaches are most apparent in the acute 'crisis' phase, when a woman first receives the diagnosis of cancer. The counsellor may provide advice and also help women to make more informed decisions about treatment options based on a knowledge about the disease and the patient's own personal circumstances. When the woman has had an opportunity to express her doubts, fears, and worries and to consider the options available to her, the skilled counsellor should offer support and encourage the woman in the development of positive coping strategies which may help the woman through her forthcoming treatment. The following example is part of a transcript from a session between a counsellor and a 48-year-old woman who had just been told that her breast lump was malignant and that she needed to have a mastectomy.

Counsellor:	Mr C. tells me that you are very upset about the prospect of having a mastectomy. Would you like to tell me more about these feelings?
Patient:	I'm just not having one; that's all. (Long pause, patient crying.)
Counsellor:	I'm sorry to see you so distressed, but it might help if you could face telling me more about your worries.
Patient:	My mother died of breast cancer and she had a mastectomy, so it didn't make any difference – I don't see the point of going through it all if you die anyway.
Counsellor:	I'm sorry to hear about your mother, but I understand how you must be feeling. There is no reason why the same thing should happen to you, although I can see why you might be worried that it will. Do you know how far advanced your mother's breast cancer was when she had her operation?
Patient:	Well, I think it was quite big – you didn't really talk about those things much in those days, so she hadn't told anyone about it.

Counsellor:	I see, so it was quite some time ago that...
Patient:	Yes, nearly 20 years ago.
Counsellor:	It might help you to concentrate on the fact that your breast cancer is actually at a very early stage. The reason Mr C. thinks that a mastectomy would be better is that the lump, although small, is very close to your nipple, and if he removed the lump and surrounding tissue you might not be very happy with the result.
Patient:	Yes, he told me all that and that I'd have to have the radium treatment as well.
Counsellor:	Do you know what that involves – coming up to the hospital for treatment every day for six weeks?
Patient:	Oh – I don't like the thought of that.
Counsellor:	What do you see as the problem?
Patient:	Well, my job for a start – we're in business, my husband and I.
Counsellor:	Has your husband come with you to see Mr C.?
Patient:	No – the business, you see. (Patient begins to cry again.)
Counsellor:	I'm sorry that you are feeling so upset – is it because of your husband? (Patient nods.)
Counsellor:	Would you like to tell me about it?
Patient:	We've not had an easy time of things lately and the business isn't going that well – we've got the shop – he doesn't need all this as well.
Counsellor:	I'm sure that things must be very difficult at the moment for small businesses with the current political situation. How do you think your husband will react to the news that you've got breast cancer?
Patient:	Oh, he'll be really upset for me. We're very close.
Counsellor:	What would he feel about the operation?
Patient:	He'd just want me to have the best treatment, whatever that is. He's marvellous you know. (Patient crying again.)
Counsellor:	That's good that he would support you – has Mr C. offered to talk to him with you?
Patient:	Oh yes, he was really kind – I must sound so ungrateful – it isn't his fault that I've got to have this thing. I know I'm being silly.

Counsellor: I don't think he would expect you to be grateful and you're not being silly. All he wants is for you to have the treatment that's right for you. He wouldn't force anything that you didn't want, you know.

Patient: What shall I do?

Counsellor: It isn't for me to tell you, but we could just go through some of the things that you've told me about yourself and some of the things that I know about the various treatments and then come to a decision.

In this particular situation the counsellor needed to establish whether or not the distress being displayed by the patient was due to any unknown factors in the woman's life. It has been shown that the values, beliefs, and perceptions (see Chapter 2) of the meanings that illnesses such as cancer have for an individual together with previous illness experiences may play an important part in determining the coping strategies employed (Lipowski 1970). Thus, several key issues, such as the death of the patient's mother from breast cancer and worries about the patient's recent business venture, were influencing the way in which she reacted to the news that she herself had breast cancer and needed a mastectomy. Bard and Sutherland (1955) were the first research workers to point out that those patients likely to fear breast cancer most of all, or delay seeking treatment were those with experience of relatives who had died of the disease. Furthermore, this poor experience usually manifested itself in women adopting a more futile or hopeless attitude towards the likely outcome of treatment than that displayed by women who knew someone who had been cured of the disease (Jamison *et al.* 1978). Fortunately, the counsellor was able to point out to the woman that her cancer was at an early stage unlike her mother's disease; thus, she was not necessarily going to share the same fate.

The counsellor was also able to provide and reinforce information given by the doctor about the technical reasons for recommending mastectomy and the pros and cons of conservative surgery with radiation therapy. This is relevant, as an understanding of the relative merits of different treatments may be extremely important in assisting the development and utilization of effective coping strategies. Individuals who feel confident about their forthcoming treatment are probably able to play a more active part in coping with therapy and fighting the disease. Furthermore, researchers such as

Moss and Schaefer (1984) have highlighted the importance of a sense of self-efficacy or mastery in the adjustment and adaptation to serious illness; consequently, involving the patient in thorough discussions about treatment and planning means of coping may be vital. This is particularly true for those women who already have a strong internal locus of control, as they are much more likely to employ problem-focused forms of coping (Anderson 1977).

The breast cancer counsellor should also be aware that some of the differences in coping strategies may be class based. Recent research has shown that people from lower socioeconomic groups who tend anyway to have a more negative self-perception and who are less self-directed may well be those patients who adopt acceptance/resignation type coping rather than confrontational or avoidance strategies (Feifel et al. 1987).

The importance of social support to overall coping in breast cancer will be discussed more fully later in this chapter. However, in the example given above the counsellor established the potential support available to the woman. In this particular case, the most significant source of emotional support was the patient's spouse, but it could be a friend, parent, sibling, lover, or child. Enlisting the help of this person and involving them in the patient's rehabilitation is crucial. Those patients without a clearly identifiable supporter or with poor supports are most at risk of developing serious psychological dysfunction and may need extra counselling help. Establishing the patient's perception of her partner's more likely reactions to the news of her breast cancer and the treatment involved can also provide clues as to her ability to cope. Some women are much more distressed about their partner's expected reaction than about their own feelings.

Another important point to notice from the transcript is the way in which the counsellor acknowledged the patient's feelings throughout and yet also managed to elicit some of the precise reasons why the woman was so upset. She was then able to provide extra information and honest reassurance. One final thing to recognize is the fact that although this counselling session involved primarily what I have described as directive and informative elements, at no stage did the counsellor attempt to tell the patient what to do. She managed both to *provide* information and to *elicit* important information which was then reflected back in an attempt to enable the patient to weigh up the advantages and disadvantages of the treatment options, given her own unique situation. Later on in this particular session the patient was able to see that mastectomy was the most appropriate surgical treatment to have and went away feeling more confident and less negative and distressed than she had at the beginning of the session.

Pre-operative counselling needs

Nearly all patients about to undergo surgery for any reason, not just breast cancer, experience a certain amount of anxiety. There is plenty of evidence to show that the pre-operative psychological preparation of patients results in fewer post-operative complications, less pain, and a shorter stay in hospital. Most lay people are rather ignorant of quite simple details concerning anaesthesia and what is involved during surgery, so good preparation may allay some of these worries. Fortunately, the distressing practice of performing a frozen section and then proceeding to mastectomy if cancer was found, is rarely necessary these days with the advent of such things as cytology (see Chapter 1). Nevertheless, some women who are admitted for breast biopsy are extremely fearful that they will regain consciousness and find that their breast has been removed. Clearly stating that this will not happen can be immensely reassuring pre-operatively.

A considerable number of women are unaware of what the chest wall looks like following a mastectomy. The counsellor can help by describing the scar or providing photographs, as the images that women may have are often worse than the reality. The following extract from an interview with a patient demonstrates this point well.

Interviewer: You told me that Miss M. was very helpful the night before your operation. Can you tell me what happened?

Patient: Well I feel a bit embarrassed about it all now really, but you see I'm not one to ask questions, doctors scare me a bit, even though Mr P. was so nice. Anyway I really didn't know what was going to happen when they cut my breast off. I thought, oh my God, what do they do – use something like a bacon-slicer. I imagined that I'd have a great raw patch where it had been like sliced off. I was so worried – anyway Miss M. asked me if there was anything that I didn't understand or wanted to ask her and, oh, I was so relieved. She said lots of women didn't know quite what to expect and offered to show me a picture. It looked far better than I'd been imagining.

Post-operative counselling needs

Immediately post-surgery

It is not unusual for women to experience euphoria post-operatively, as the following quotation from a 56-year-old woman who had a mastectomy shows.

> I can't say that I honestly had much pain, although my arm was very stiff – I felt great – it felt as though a great weight had been lifted off my head. I felt almost drunk with relief that they had got rid of my breast and all the cancer. I'd been having nightmares the two weeks before the operation thinking about cancer spreading everywhere. I felt so happy that it had gone, I really felt like I was – well – *alive* again.

The women who experience these euphoric reactions need counselling help as they are often the women who later become severely depressed and pessimistic about their future.

During the period from discovery of the lump, through to hearing the diagnosis and then having the operation, a woman's thoughts may be so centred on coping with what she sees as an immediate threat to life, and then physical recovery from the operation, that she does not have either the time or the emotional energy to consider the more long-term implications of what has happened. Paradoxically, when a woman first returns home and starts to feel physically better she may start to feel emotionally worse; worries about things such as recurrence, body image, or the reaction of her partner to her breast cancer treatment may start to surface.

> I was great while I was in hospital – there were lots of laughs and the staff-nurses and doctors were all so kind, but I've been rock-bottom since I got home. I kept bursting into tears for no real reason and to think I didn't shed a tear while I was in. I was so relieved after the operation that it was all over, but it's not is it? It's all just starting – I'm still a cancer patient. I don't feel

very sure any more that things will be okay. I keep feeling my breast wondering if they got all the cancer. I keep thinking maybe I should have had it all taken away. I was glad that they didn't do a mastectomy at the time, but I'll never be sure that it was the right thing to do. My GP told me I should think myself lucky, so I haven't told him how depressed I am.

During radiotherapy or chemotherapy treatment

I mentioned in Chapter 4 that those women 'lucky enough' to have surgery that conserves the breast need just as much counselling support as those who have a mastectomy (Fallowfield *et al.* 1987). Such women still have to cope with the knowledge that they have cancer and must also endure further treatment such as radiotherapy. Unfortunately, the limited resources available in many of our hospitals mean that only crisis counselling is available for the most obviously distressed women and an incorrect assumption is made that women who have breast-conserving surgery are less likely to require the services of a counsellor. All women with breast cancer, however this may be treated, should be given the opportunity of counselling support post-operatively.

In Chapter 4 I mentioned some of the psychological problems that can occur during radiotherapy and this is a time when informative and supportive counselling can be extremely valuable, especially if the counsellor can allay some of the fears that radiotherapy is harmful. An example can be seen in the following comments made by a woman who suffered from severe anxiety during her treatment.

I was really frightened during the radium treatment. They didn't really tell me much about it and they were always so busy that I didn't like to be a trouble, but I just got more and more worried. You hear all these things about people getting leukaemia from radiation and I thought that if anyone touched me I might contaminate them. I didn't pick up my granddaughter during the treatment. I bumped into the breast nurse who had seen me at the beginning and she sat me down and asked me how things were going. I only wish I'd been to see her earlier, as she explained everything and convinced me that it was safe. I found it much easier to cope after that.

Those women who require chemotherapy may also value the support of a counsellor, especially if he or she has had training in behavioural techniques, such as desensitization and anxiety management (Burish and Lyles 1981). Drug therapy which includes anti-emetics and anxiolytics may help to a certain extent with the nausea and vomiting experienced by the majority of patients during chemotherapy sessions. However, Chapter 4 described the problems that a significant number of women (between 25 to 65 per cent) experience with anticipatory nausea and vomiting. These distressing side effects may need behavioural interventions as well as drugs. Cella *et al.* (1986) have shown that the sights and smells reminding cured individuals of their chemotherapy sessions may still elicit nausea and vomiting *ten years* after the cessation of treatment. At particular risk of developing adverse conditioned responses to chemotherapy are those patients who are anxious about having such treatment (Van Komen and Redd 1985). Thus, relieving patients of their anxiety with effective, informative counselling, together with such techniques as passive relaxation through hypnosis with imagery (Redd *et al.* 1982), could be seen as a vital prophylactic part of treatment.

Many women also find that alopecia can further damage their self-image during chemotherapy, especially if mastectomy has already caused a major assault to body image or if the cosmetic appearance of a conserved breast is less than good. In a study reporting the side effects of patients undergoing 30 different chemotherapy regimens 84 per cent thought that alopecia was the most distressing symptom (Penman *et al.* 1984). The counsellor may help women with appropriate psychological preparation for hair loss. Again, informative and supportive counselling is needed so that women are not surprised or frightened when their hair starts to fall out. Reassurance that hair will grow back is important, as is encouragement to get a good, well-fitting wig made prior to hair loss.

Another assault to a fragile body image made worse by surgery and alopecia is the weight gain seen in women receiving adjuvant hormonal therapy such as megestrol acetate for metastatic breast cancer (Knobf 1986). Counselling aimed at promoting self-esteem and self-confidence is very necessary at this time.

It should be fairly obvious by now that confrontational, cathartic, catalytic, and supportive counselling are all very relevant during chemotherapy. Women may feel so physically awful that worries about death re-emerge or they may even consider death to be a more attractive proposition than having to endure further courses of chemotherapy. Patients may also experience a strong sense of having lost control, thus the primary role of the counsellor again may be confrontational and catalytic in an attempt to help women regain a sense of control and to stop them feeling so negative about themselves and the outcome of treatment. The description of chemotherapy given below by a woman in her early 30s illustrates these issues well.

Nothing that has ever happened to me in my life before could have prepared me for that experience. One moment I was well, happy, successful, and reasonably attractive and within the space of six weeks I'd learned that I had cancer, I'd lost part of my breast, most of my hair, and my whole life revolved around either feeling or being sick. I couldn't believe that I would ever get better or look better again. I felt that my life had already ended. I couldn't even think straight or make a simple decision. Fortunately my sister put me in touch with a psychologist friend of hers who helped me to relax properly – I had become so anxious about being sick that that in itself made me sick. She also helped me feel more positive about the future – she helped me feel that I *had* a future if I wanted one.

Post-treatment counselling needs

By the time three months has elapsed since their surgery, most women with breast cancer have finished their radiotherapy, although courses of chemotherapy may continue for much longer. The reactions of women when treatment has finished are difficult to predict and vary between individuals. As I have shown in previous chapters, some women suffer anxiety and depression which does not remit of its own accord. Hence those women who experience psychological problems in the early part of their treatment should not be abandoned to work out their difficulties alone. Given the scarcity of adequate counselling services it may be important to try and identify those women with potentially inadequate or maladaptive coping strategies for more long-term help. Penman (1982) found that women who employed a variety of what she described as 'tackling' behaviours combined with mastery, rationalizing, and reinterpretive strategies early on, displayed better coping and were less distressed at four months post-surgery, than those women who made use of capitulating or avoidance strategies at the outset.

One interesting and seemingly paradoxical finding is that, despite the disturbing side effects, women who complete their chemotherapy may become extremely anxious and frightened instead of delighted as one might expect.

Interviewer: How did you feel when you finished your final course of chemotherapy?

Patient: You may find this difficult to believe after all I've said about the problems I had, but I was absolutely terrified. During the chemo I kept myself going by thinking about the fact that I was being so sick because it was working. Well, when I finished, instead of being really pleased I was scared that the cancer cells would, like, start growing again.

This type of reaction is also common in some women whom one might suppose would be pleased when told by their surgeon that the frequency of follow-up visits and monitoring can decrease from three monthly to six monthly or yearly. The need for reassurance that all is well continues for several years. Meyerowitz *et al.* (1983) found that at least 37 per cent of women two years after the completion of their adjuvant chemotherapy said that they needed reassurance that all was still well and felt worried that the cancer might return without further chemotherapy. Likewise, Holland *et al.* (1979) showed that patients exhibited a rise in anxiety at the end of radiotherapy treatment which they put down to the separation from staff whom patients felt had been exercising a surveillance over their cancer. The absence of this reassuring monitoring following the cessation of radiotherapy made women anxious that their cancer would recur. Counselling patients to expect an increase in anxiety and offering them an opportunity to discuss their worries may be of benefit.

Social support

Counsellors and other professionals with counselling skills are in short supply. Thus, most women have to rely on the help of others outside a medical setting. Although many women are able to marshal support from their family and friends and some report that love and understanding from their spouse or most significant other has increased since having cancer (Dunkel-Schetter 1984), this is by no means true for every woman. Peters-Golden (1982) found in her sample of 100 women with breast cancer that over one half (52 per cent) felt that people avoided or feared them, 14 per cent felt 'pitied' and 72 per cent felt misunderstood. Only 3 per cent thought that people were 'nicer' to them. These findings may seem strange to those of us who see women with breast cancer as innocent victims, but they fit in with the 'just-world' hypothesis described by Lerner and Miller (1978). Several studies show that innocent victims of a variety of things, from rape to mugging or illness, are often derogated or devalued because people tend to subscribe to a belief that the world is a fair place in which the majority of people get their just desserts. Although women with cancer may recognize that their problems evoke sympathy and pity in many people they may also detect avoidance behaviours in others who consciously or unconsciously blame the victim in some way for her own misfortune.

It comes as no surprise that women with breast cancer, caught in the middle of this ambiguous and negative social feedback, may find that their self-esteem and self-confidence withers. All of this serves to compound their feelings of depression and worthlessness. Such a situation poses the counsellor with a rather difficult problem, as it is impossible to change the attitudes and beliefs of society overnight. Nevertheless, with careful confrontational and constant supportive counselling, it may well be possible to encourage more positive thinking and self-esteem that is not dependent on social feedback from others.

The counsellor may also be able to fulfil one of the cathartic roles usually provided by spouses, friends, and relatives, that of providing the women with an opportunity to off-load feelings and fears. Even the setting of a research interview, using a semi-structured psychiatric interview, may provide some cathartic release (Fallowfield *et al.* 1987). The following extract is from a 67-year-old woman with breast cancer who wrote at the end of a research project saying:

> The real purpose of writing this letter is to thank you very much
> for your visits. I know that they are to help you with your
> research programme, but you have no idea how comforting it is

to have these visits at intervals; a real booster to the confidence, having someone spending so much time with us 'guinea pigs'.

Asking a woman if she has a confidante is a useful indicator as to how much emotional support is available to her from others. This is important, as the presence of good emotional support is so crucial to successful long-term adjustment in breast cancer. Several studies have shown strong correlations between the perception of social support and adjustment, e.g., Bloom (1982), Funch and Mettlin (1982). However, mere availability of support is not in itself sufficient, as women must also possess the ability to elicit and utilize support. There is a complex interplay between social support, sense of control, coping, and adaptation to cancer (Ell *et al.* 1989). Those women who lack appropriate support may be the people upon which to concentrate most of our scanty counselling resources.

Advanced cancer

Some of the psychological reactions of women with advanced breast cancer have already been described in Chapter 5. Counselling at this stage of the disease involves helping patients to enhance the quality of their remaining life by maximizing the use of positive coping strategies. Helping women to enjoy as much of their lives as possible can be achieved by restructuring goals, challenging negative thinking, and permitting the expression of anger, frustration, and fear. One of the difficulties confronting many women for whom death is now inevitable is the social obligation to face their demise bravely. The battlefield metaphor is used constantly in cancer with expressions such as 'fighting spirit', or she 'fought courageously' or 'she lost the battle with cancer after a brave fight'. Such a portrayal of dying from breast cancer can make some patients feel hopelessly inadequate, as the following quotation reveals.

Everyone keeps telling me that I've got to fight it, as though I've got some real chance of making things better. Well, that's all very well for them to say, but they haven't got to do it have they? I sometimes feel as though I'm letting the side down and making *them* feel bad because I don't feel like fighting – what have I got to fight for? I wish they would just let me be – I'm not scared of dying any more, but I do wish they could stop making me feel guilty about not wanting to fight. It's been difficult enough coming to terms with having this wretched cancer, without having to be made to feel that I'm a weak and cowardly person for not fitting in with their plans as to how I should die.

The work of Greer and his colleagues (1979) showing (in a small sample of women) that adoption of a strategy labelled 'fighting spirit' seemed to enhance survival, has provided the rationale for counselling or therapy aimed at encouraging this coping strategy. In fact, women in the original sample of Greer *et al.* who adopted denial as their primary coping strategy also did rather better in survival terms, but one hears very little about any efforts to help sustain women who use this form of coping.

It is difficult to see how encouraging women who are approaching death to adopt strategies which they have never used previously in coping with life's crises could do anything but diminish the quality of their lives.

Counselling case study

I have tried to provide different examples of the sort of counselling that women with breast cancer may require at different stages of their disease. Unfortunately, much of the counselling which takes place in our busy under-resourced health service is crisis counselling or casualty-based rather than prophylactic (see Table 6.2). In the case history that follows I describe the counselling support offered to one young woman from the time of her recurrent breast cancer to her eventual death. I had been asked by a consultant surgeon as a favour to visit a patient of his who was refusing an operation for recurrent breast disease.

Table 6.2 Counselling in breast cancer

Prophylactic (the ideal)	Casualty based (the reality)
anticipatory	reactive
integrated with other disciplines	not integrated
planned, scheduled	random
all clients, no 'ticket' needed	'casualties' only
Objective: to prevent or ameliorate stress and dysfunction	*Objective:* to assist patients experiencing psychological distress

Based on Nichols 1989

Maureen was a 35-year-old nurse, unmarried and living alone. Two years previously she had been diagnosed as having an inflammatory adeno-carcinoma of the right breast. After a great deal of discussion with the surgeon of her choice (being a theatre sister she was in a good position to assess the relative skills of the surgeons she worked with) and a radiotherapist, it was decided that radiotherapy and chemotherapy were the most appropriate treatments.

She tolerated the initial radiotherapy well, but had a very bad time with the side effects of chemotherapy, suffering the miseries of nausea and vomiting and losing all her hair. A year later, however, the treatment appeared to have produced a good remission of symptoms and she was able to return to work. One week prior to the request for my visit, she had discovered another lump in the affected breast. The surgeon and radiotherapist decided that the only palliative treatment likely to produce any relief and to prevent the almost certain breakdown of her chest wall was a radical mastectomy with a large latissimus dorsae skin flap and split skin grafts. She was well aware of the necessity for the operation if there was to be any chance of local control of the cancer, and had agreed to the operation. Unfortunately, a few days later she had exhibited several hysterical outbursts at work. I was asked to see her at her home. She had decided not to have any further treatment.

When I saw her Maureen was clearly very anxious and confused by her own ambivalent feelings towards the many people trying to help her. This ambivalence demonstrated itself constantly during the interview. She acknowledged embarrassment at the various hysterical outbursts that she had experienced during that week. She wanted people to ask her how she was, but then got angry and upset at them asking her, e.g., 'Why do they ask, when they know what I'm going through? or 'Fancy Dr X. or Nurse Y. not even bothering to ask or say that they are sorry'. Maureen felt utterly bewildered by the events taking place around her. She felt out of control and confused by her emotions. When asked why she had decided to decline an operation, she said that she had not actually made that decision yet. We explored the myriad of feelings that she was currently experiencing, which included fear, fatalism, and stoic acceptance. It was also apparent that she was extremely angry. When confronted with this, she cried and admitted that she felt 'cheated'. 'It isn't fair, after all that I've gone through already.' We talked about these feelings at length and it became clear that she had been trying to exert some authority and get some redress for the unfairness by refusing the operation. She felt that she had paid such a heavy price for a 'cure' with the chemotherapy and the radiotherapy and they had no right to ask more from her. She admitted that this was both an understandable and illogical response.

Maureen seemed much more forthcoming and able to articulate her other fears after admitting to these feelings; in particular, she revealed a professional abhorrence of mastectomy – she said that she had never witnessed one without feeling 'God, I hope that's never me'. She then said that she was grateful that Mr C. was doing the operation and that Dr Y. would give the anaesthetic. In contrast to some comments made at the start of our interview, demonstrating how emotionally labile she was, Maureen then pronounced total, unrealistic faith in the ability of her surgeon to 'get me well again'.

At the end of an hour-long session Maureen said that she felt much calmer and more relaxed and that she would appreciate further counselling after the operation. She asked to see me before surgery if possible. She agreed that I should telephone her doctor and let him know that she would like to talk to him again, as she now felt prepared to go ahead with the operation.

Following day

I arrived at hospital to discover that Maureen had been heavily sedated at her own request, so I was unable to talk to her. The surgeon said that she had said the counselling session had helped her a great deal.

One day post-op

I had a very short interview with Maureen, who looked very relaxed, but slightly euphoric. She claimed to have no knowledge about the day of operation and had effectively repressed everything which we had discussed the week before. She talked about going home as soon as possible, now that 'everything was fine'.

Three days post-op

I received a telephone call from sister in charge of the ward. Maureen was very distressed, oscillating between no communication at all to tearful outbursts. She looked very sad and tearful when I arrived. She said that she was very angry that the surgeon had been 'so cruel'. When asked to expand, she revealed that when the dressing had been removed he joked about the skin flap and had said 'That's your back you're looking at'. She felt upset and let down that he should have joked and was cross that he had caused her so much pain. She said that she felt like 'chucking the towel in – I just can't take any more. I wish I hadn't agreed to go through with all this'. She said that she wished to return to last week when she had still had a choice. I pointed out that, according to her, last week had actually been hell, and that the freedom to choose between having an operation or not had not been a comfortable situation for her. I suggested that this choice was in fact an illusion and such retrospection was in fact a displacement activity for getting on with the real business of adjusting to what *is*, not what was, or what might have been.

Following more emotional disclosures, Maureen appeared to be emerging from her attitude of 'poor me'. However, she was adamant that she would not undergo any more treatment and expressed profound hostility towards the surgeon who had 'brought this all on her'. She requested another visit from me the next day.

Four days post-op

Maureen was much calmer and wanted to talk about some of the issues contributing to her emotional lability. She said that she felt guilty about having been so angry with the surgeon whom she actually admired a great deal. She acknowledged that she felt extremely grateful much of the time for his understanding and sympathy. She seemed helped by a discussion on the apparent necessity for her to attribute blame and hostility somewhere for all the distress that her illness was causing her.

She admitted to feeling 'very frightened' about her future and that being angry about events or with someone stopped her feeling so scared. She recognized that she needed some help with the difficult feelings that she was experiencing. For example, she felt that people close to her were not demonstrating that they cared enough or that they could not readily sympathize with her plight. She was particularly angry with other medical or nursing colleagues, who kept telling her that everything would be all right. Maureen had not thought about the possibility that some of her friends and relatives were just as upset as she was about her problems. We discussed the possibility that the only way in which they could cope was by denial or focusing on other things and that this could well be interpreted as indifference by Maureen. She also talked about a male friend whom she had asked to leave after he had been visiting for only ten minutes on the grounds that she was too upset to talk to him. When he got up to leave, she became quite irrational and hysterical. 'I only told him to go because I wanted him to stay! He failed the test; he didn't care.'

Ten days post-op

Maureen was rather withdrawn and claimed that she did not want to talk about herself. (Was this another test similar to the one her friend had 'failed')? Ten minutes later she managed to express her deep anxieties about her prognosis (which was poor for this type of breast cancer). We discussed the options available to her which were to carry on working for as long as possible, or to stop work and do all the things that she 'had always dreamt of doing'. She then decided that work was actually her life. It provided her with a sense of purpose and importance and was her only real social opportunity. She said 'If I do give up work, I'll just curl up in a heap and die.'

Twenty-one days post-op

Maureen was discharged home. She asked to see me in a month's time.

One month later

Maureen looked quite well and relaxed. She said that she had done a lot of thinking over the past few weeks and could face whatever was ahead more constructively. She did not have any hostility left towards her doctors, but still was experiencing periods of 'Why me?' She said that counselling had been a great help.

Maureen had required immediate crisis counselling. She had to cope with an iniquitous, unpleasant, anxiety-provoking situation, enough to stretch even the most psychologically robust individual. Her sorry predicament exposed the limitations of her personal coping repertoire. Having exhausted all the strategies available to her she felt overwhelmed by feelings of inadequacy, stress, and loss of autonomy. From a counselling point of view, she required help in facing up to the reality of the crisis; this involved help in discouraging denial and promotion of some objectivity in her thinking about the situation. This was partially achieved by breaking up the crisis into more manageable doses. False reassurance was being provided by well-meaning friends; Maureen seemed to be helped more by the counsellor encouraging her to discuss the reality of her plight. Post-operatively Maureen needed a great deal of help in dealing with problems of projection and hostility, and this was especially apparent in her need to find someone to 'blame' for everything.

One year later

I was asked to see Maureen again by her GP and she herself telephoned requesting a visit. When I arrived she was very distressed and weepy and full of complaints about the dreadful way in which everyone was treating her, in particular the radiotherapist and anaesthetist who ran a pain clinic. After she had off-loaded her primary criticisms, we discussed the rank order of things that were upsetting her most. She had in fact recently learned that she had metastatic disease and had returned to her old need to blame someone – in this case the radiotherapist who broke the news to her. She was very angry that his treatment had not worked and very concerned about her appearance. (Steroid therapy had made her gain two to three stone in weight.) Maureen acknowledged that this bad news had sparked off all the original feelings of anger, blame, and hurt that no one cared enough. We discussed the possibility that she was making it very difficult for her friends and colleagues to show her how much they cared, by her own behaviour. She accepted that whatever they did she was critical and complaining and we talked about ways in which she could view their actions in a more positive light. She then commented that she was most angry about the fact that they were all well and alive and that she was dying. She still viewed the fact of her breast cancer as grossly unfair in that many of her colleagues were far less deserving of their good health.

Maureen died approximately two months later. She was still very angry with the world, but kept insisting that counselling had made her view things differently and had helped. I have already mentioned in previous chapters that women with a strong sense of 'Why me?'

who subscribe to a just-world hypothesis are very difficult to counsel. In the event, Maureen claimed that she had been helped even though that might not have been apparent to her long-suffering friends and medical carers.

Does counselling in breast cancer work?

Most women with breast cancer attest to the benefits of receiving counselling at some stage during their treatment.

The following extract is from another letter sent to me by a woman with breast cancer who was deemed to be so depressed and anxious during a research project that we decided to solicit counselling help for her.

> I thought that you might like to know that I have had four really good months thanks to my counsellor who has really helped me to think positively and to learn to really relax and gain confidence in myself again. I really feel fine – the best I've ever felt since I had my operation three years ago. Thank you for all the help you have given me – I do hope your project will enable more people to have expert counselling.

However, not everyone needs counselling. Indeed, there may be a few women who find that such an intervention is either too intrusive or that it hampers the natural course of their emotional adjustment; other women may feel that they have adequate support from other sources and sufficient inner coping abilities; occasionally patients may reject counselling on the grounds that it is only for 'mad' people. One patient told me that she did not wish to talk about her breast cancer to a psychologist.

> I really don't know why Mr H. asked you to see me – I'm not mad you know. If it's all the same to you, I'd like to keep my thoughts and problems to myself.

Nevertheless, anyone who works with women with breast cancer can see that for the majority skilled counselling appears to make a great difference in both the short-and long-term adjustment process. Unfortunately, scientific evidence for the efficacy of counselling is rather thin. At best most evaluation studies show that whilst counselling may not prevent such things as anxiety and depression, regular contact and monitoring by a breast nurse counsellor, who may refer patients on to a liaison psychiatrist if necessary, may ameliorate or reduce psychiatric morbidity (Maguire *et al.* 1980). Another study reporting a small and transiently favourable outcome was that by Watson *et al.* (1988), who randomized forty consecutive breast cancer patients to either routine care or routine care and counselling from a specialist nurse. The nurse counsellor offered mainly informative and directive counselling as she was responsible for fitting the breast prosthesis, but she also provided crisis intervention counselling on demand. The only significant difference between the counselled and non-counselled group of women occurred at three months, when depression and a sense of loss of control was less for those women who had counselling, but by twelve months these differences had disappeared.

There is also some, fairly controversial, evidence suggesting that counselling women with breast cancer improves survival. For example, Spiegel *et al.* (1989) in a prospective study, looked at the survival outcome in eighty-three women with metastatic breast cancer randomized to supportive group counselling and self-hypnosis or standard care. They found a significant survival advantage to the counselled group. However, these data have been criticized on the grounds that, with such a small sample, other variables may have influenced outcome.

There are many methodological reasons why evaluation studies may fail to show any real benefit to women given counselling: they often have small patient samples; the outcome measure(s) used, such as clinical anxiety and/or depression, may be too gross to pick up important but subtle changes between groups; what counts as counselling may be rather vaguely defined; and the person doing the counselling may lack the necessary skills. This is a potentially serious problem, as counselling is obviously only as good as the person doing it. Counselling that works in one institution may fail in another if the beneficial effects are so dependent on the skill, training, and supervision of the counsellor. Fallowfield and Roberts (1992) conducted a national survey of oncology counsellors and specialist cancer nurses and found that few had any formal training qualifications. For a good comprehensive review of the literature looking at evaluative studies of counselling in cancer, the interested reader should try either Watson (1983) or the more recent review by Cunningham (1988). Both of these articles discuss other methodological reasons (which are beyond the scope of this book) as to why it is so difficult to demonstrate a clear benefit from counselling.

Trying to identify, at an early stage, the areas of psychosocial and sexual life that are causing women concern and then applying specific interventions may be of more value than attempting to give somewhat unstructured counselling to all women.

Who should do the counselling?

Volunteers

I have already described in other chapters examples of poor counselling, which far from helping the unfortunate patient may actually have made a sorry situation even worse. These examples were taken from interviews with women who had received counselling from both professionally employed counsellors and volunteers. Discussions as to who is best placed to be an effective counsellor, can cause considerable controversy. Volunteer counsellors, especially those who have been 'victims' of breast cancer, may well be able to offer their fellow sufferers a form of experiential empathy that few of us fortunate enough to have avoided breast cancer could ever hope to emulate. This personal sensitivity to the problems of having had a life-threatening disease and coping with the treatments is however a unique experience; each individual, whilst sharing some common reactions and insights, has her own personal history, social and sexual relationships, occupational commitments, future plans, dreams and expectations, and so forth, which ultimately affect and have an impact upon the adjustment and coping strategies employed. Too often, therefore, these idiosyncratic factors may interfere with attempts to help another woman with her problems. Furthermore, many potential 'victim-counsellors' have as their primary motivation either an acknowledged or maybe subconscious desire to understand more of their own experiences by trying to help others – Reissman's so-called helper-therapy principle (1965). Such women need to be actively discouraged from counselling for their own protection as well as that of others (Mantell 1983; Fallowfield 1988). It can be very distressing, unless one has considerable skill and training, to get too close to the emotional difficulties that a woman with breast cancer may be experiencing. When this happens to someone who shares the same diagnosis, it can be particularly destructive and damaging. At the very least victim-counsellors should be given supportive supervision if they are to be effective; they should also be people who have managed to cope well with their own cancer, be emotionally stable, and display good communication skills, especially good listening skills (Mastrovito *et al.* 1989).

Support groups

As one-to-one counselling for everyone with breast cancer who needs it is too labour intensive for our under-resourced health service to provide, many patients, their relatives, and friends have started support groups. These may be professionally led by a trained counsellor, nurse, or social worker or they may be organized by the patients and families themselves. Some support groups feel that the presence of professionals limits the spontaneity of the group and many clinicians have concerns that much damage from misinformation can be caused. Opinions are mixed. One woman with breast cancer told me that she found the experience distressing as the group tended to attract only those people who were coping rather poorly, or who had a great deal of anger and dissatisfaction with their medical carers to off-load. Conversely, another woman told me:

> I only went along twice, there were several women there who seemed to have had none of the difficulties that I had. They were all making jokes about their false boobs and so on. I found it all rather upsetting. They made me feel odd, like I wasn't coping very well.

Plant *et al.* (1987) evaluated a support group for a mixed group of cancer patients, their families, and friends. They reported that only 18 per cent of people invited to the group came and that reasons given for *not* coming included:

> satisfaction that all questions had already been answered (56 per cent), difficulties with distance and/or transport (50 per cent), a desire to forget about cancer (37 per cent), a dislike of group discussions (25 per cent), and a fear that hearing about other people's problems would be depressing (19 per cent).

The authors concluded, however, that the majority of those patients who did attend benefited from sharing their experiences with others.

Conclusion

It seems fair to say that counselling provision is necessary to help ameliorate the distress provoked by the diagnosis of cancer. It may be useful in assisting the patient to make informed decisions about treatment options. It may be of value to patients' families and friends and can assist them in providing the stable, effective social support necessary to enhance coping and adjustment. It can possibly enhance survival.

Unfortunately, we have too few properly trained oncology counsellors. Many of the specialist nurses employed tackle too great a patient load and work with little support or supervision (Roberts and Fallowfield 1990). Instead of being able to offer an ideal *prophylactic* service (see Table 6.2), the reality is a *casualty*-based system offering mainly crisis counselling.

Chapter seven

Conclusion and new directions

The guiding principle is respect for persons, which means that competent patients have the right to know and to decide. ... Consent that is not informed is not valid; it does not give clinicians a right to proceed with diagnostic or therapeutic procedures.

(Schoene-Seifert and Childress 1986)

There is still no consensus as to the most appropriate way in which to treat the 24,500 women who develop breast cancer in the United Kingdom each year. Despite the large sums of money spent on research throughout the world, a really major breakthrough in terms of cure still eludes us. There is no firm evidence that different surgical policies increase survival and the value of adjuvant radiotherapy and/or chemotherapy for some women remains uncertain. Two things at least are clear. First, there are few topics that arouse so much controversy among clinicians. Second, this background of uncertainty does little to inspire hope and confidence in those women unfortunate enough to receive a diagnosis of breast cancer. If the supposed experts cannot agree then how can a woman make a truly informed decision about treatment options?

In the face of increasing demands made for more patient autonomy, the plight of the woman with breast cancer provides an interesting example of the dilemmas involved. When discussing this issue, I am well aware that my own opinions would probably be rejected by many who, from the comfort of their own armchairs, confidently espouse the view that:

1 all women must *always* be given a choice of treatment;

2   if given such a choice *all* women invariably would choose
    lumpectomy over mastectomy; and
3   choice in itself would prevent most of the psychological
    distress described throughout this book.

Unfortunately things are rarely that simple. As someone who has
worked with all sorts of women with breast cancer over the past
twenty-two years, I lack the firm conviction of the armchair or dinner
party experts who feel that there is only one correct way to handle the
situation and that, furthermore, this method is appropriate for all
women. Issuing dogmatic statements as to what should take place
during a consultation which is almost bound to be fraught with difficulties about the benefits of different management policies, is
misguided, if not plain silly. Those who hypothesize from afar appear
to assume that women are a somewhat homogeneous group who will all
have similar responses and reactions. Working with women who have
breast cancer quickly teaches one that they are heterogeneous, thus
an approach that benefits some may singularly fail to help others.

My knowledge about the attitudes and emotions breast cancer
sufferers experience is based on my work with them as a nurse, as a
counsellor, and finally as a research psychologist. In these various
capacities I have witnessed first-hand and listened to many patients'
accounts of their consultations with surgeons who have widely
differing styles. These styles may range from old-style paternalism to
what might be described as modern-day clinical glasnost. Following
their consultations, I have interviewed women about their feelings. It
is surprisingly difficult to predict those who will be deeply distressed
or those who will feel reassured and comforted by these different
styles of consulting as I shall illustrate in the examples which follow.

Despite the stereotypical portrayal of breast cancer surgeons as
somewhat insensitive and sadistic, I have seen many caring and
compassionate surgeons (who are more numerous than popular
myth suggests) attempt to describe to women what is known about
breast cancer and the options available to them in terms of surgery
and adjuvant therapy. Such consultations with women encouraged to
play a major role in the decision-making process might be viewed as
the ideal, the kind of good practice that all should be working
towards. But what do patients experience as a result? Reactions are
not as uniformly positive as the advocates of patient autonomy
would suggest. The majority of women are appreciative and grateful

for the opportunity to make the decision for themselves, like this woman who said:

> I must say that I was rather surprised but very pleased when he asked me which operation I preferred. He didn't hurry me and told me that it would be perfectly alright for me to go home and think about it a bit more. He encouraged me to talk to my husband about it. He also gave me a booklet from BACUP that explained all the treatments. I hadn't realised that there would be alternatives. I'd rather assumed that I'd just be told that I'd have to have a mastectomy and that would be that.

However, other women may feel quite bewildered and distressed if asked to make a decision as the following quotation shows.

> When he asked me what I wanted him to do I was very upset. I mean he's meant to be the expert isn't he? How should I be expected to know what's the best if he doesn't. I thought it was cruel, I didn't know what to say. I asked him what he would do if it was his wife's X-ray and tests in front of him and he just said that what mattered was what I wanted. I don't think it's fair to say that to people like me who don't know much about illness and operations. In the end, I just asked my daughter who used to be a nurse what I should do.

Perhaps an increase in education about health matters may result in lay people feeling more confident about decision-making so that women who exhibit the reaction seen in the last example will become much rarer. However, at the moment a significant minority are unhappy about being asked to choose. True autonomy and respect for women's rights should surely include their right to decline the offer to make their own decision. Katz (1984) describes this as an expression of 'psychological autonomy' with an informed patient opting not to make medical decisions, preferring instead to authorize the doctor to make all decisions about treatment on their behalf. This seems a more acceptable proposition than forcing participation in decision-making on a reluctant patient and it does mean the clinician is still expected to provide information. But do all women necessarily want full information? Below is an illustration of what might be termed caring paternalism and it provides an example of a category of patient who merely wants reassurance, not information or participation. This rather elderly woman told me:

> I was very upset when he told me that it was a bit more serious than mastitis, but he held my hand and said 'just you let me do all the worrying for you, we'll have you in for a few more tests next week and then I'll do whatever is best to clear this problem up'. He really was so kind, I had every confidence that everything would be alright.

Such a paternalistic approach, quite rightly, would enrage many, but some women undoubtedly do respond very positively to this style of consulting. The problem comes when doctors expect that all patients should be prepared to exhibit such uninformed, unconditional acceptance and confidence in their clinical judgement. It clearly would not suit the patient in the next example who was the victim of the most patronizing chauvinism and disrespect.

> He just said, 'Don't worry my dear, it's a growth, but we'll have it off for you next week.' I said, 'Have what off, just the lump or my whole breast?' He looked at the nurse and the young doctor with him with this really pained expression and then asked me if I'd been reading the *Guardian* or something. He gave me no useful information, just this bland reassurance that everything would be all right if I just trusted him! I was furious and made my GP send me to see someone else. As it happened, I ended up having a mastectomy anyway, but at least I understood why. In my case, with the tumour being so close to the nipple, and having rather small breasts anyway, the second surgeon said that he'd recommend mastectomy. At least I *felt* as though I'd been given some say in the matter.

This last point in the quotation above deserves more attention. What the majority of patients really want is more information as to why different policies are being pursued, rather than more autonomy in determining their treatment. There is some experimental evidence suggesting that this is certainly the case as far as cancer is concerned (Cassileth *et al.* 1980; Sutherland *et al.* 1989). In the latter study 62 per cent of patients with cancer who displayed very high information-seeking behaviour, nevertheless wished to have little or no involvement in the actual decision-making.

Research examining the influence that patient choice might have on psychological adjustment in breast cancer specifically, is sparse and generally methodologically flawed. For example, two studies published in the United Kingdom involved very small samples of women and a short follow-up (Ashcroft *et al.* 1985; Morris *et al.* 1989). Thus, the assertion that choosing treatment will necessarily lead to a decline in psychiatric morbidity cannot be substantiated yet from published research data. A study currently being conducted with a three-year follow-up might soon provide more data in this important issue (Fallowfield *et al.* 1990).

One of the reasons why we need to gather more information about the long-term implications that encouraging women to assume responsibility for their treatment may have on psychological adjustment, concerns the problem of women assuming responsibility for having chosen 'wrongly'. This may be particularly true in the case of those women who opt for breast-conserving procedures. If things go well for a woman who has played a major role in determining her surgical treatment then there may be no problem, but most of the advocates of breast-conserving procedures forget the psychological distress produced by locally recurring disease. Estimates vary but breast cancer recurs in approximately 20 per cent of women treated by lumpectomy (Locker *et al.* 1989).

There are some reports in the literature describing the damaging psychological impact of patients assuming responsibility for unsuccessful treatment outcomes (Clements and Sider 1983). However, evidence from other areas of medicine suggests that certain adaptive cognitive behaviours may be developed to relieve cognitive dissonance. Thus, patients are protected from too much self-recrimination following a 'failed' treatment decision (Wagener and Taylor 1986). As far as breast cancer is concerned, it could well be that many women anticipate the regret which they might experience for a bad decision, and are therefore reluctant to participate actively in decision-making and prefer to return this responsibility to the surgeon (see also Hershey and Baron 1987).

None of my arguments should be interpreted as a suggestion that difficult, ambiguous, and confusing information about breast cancer should be withheld from women or that those patients who wish to take a very active role in decision-making should be discouraged. I am merely attempting to present some of the arguments made in support of different attitudes to patient autonomy and, more importantly, to reflect the experience of women who have actually been through the trauma of a consultation about their diagnosis and how it should be treated. Too often this important topic gets clouded by irrational polemic. Some people appear determined to see surgeons as autocrats of the worst kind, unwilling to relinquish their role of omnipotence. While there are plenty of clinicians reluctant to acknowledge that patients could be equal partners in the decision-making process, or who feel that their professionalism is threatened by any suggestion of more patient autonomy; there are others who quite genuinely believe that providing patients with too much information about the uncertainty surrounding different treatments and making them participate in decision-making, is psychologically damaging if not unethical. None of this does much to help the unfortunate woman caught in the middle.

No one in this debate can claim to be on the side of the angels. We need much more rigorous research on the subject. This might lead to better training in appropriate communication skills for doctors dealing with patients with cancer. Improvements in basic health education for patients are needed, so that people are less confused about medical information and, consequently, may feel a little less intimidated about asking questions. Maybe in the interim more use should be made of nurses, psychologists, and others trained in patient advocacy. All these measures could relieve patients of some of their anxiety during consultations and help them to feel more informed. Only then can the real issues in the debate about choice become a little clearer.

Conclusion

The majority of people who discover that they have cancer, irrespective of the site involved, experience considerable fear and distress. Some of this anxiety might be alleviated if the treatments currently available were less toxic and more effective. Arguments about the most appropriate therapeutic modalities in breast cancer will continue, but secure data from properly-conducted randomized trials of different treatments may emerge before the end of this century. One of the many hopes for the future is that, with improved knowledge, the need for surgery will disappear altogether and that research to develop pharmacological means of selectively destroying breast cancer cells, without causing damaging toxicity to other normal cells will succeed. We also need to find better methods than radiographic mammography for detecting the disease at a stage when treatment is likely to be of most benefit. Hopefully we may also be able to make some advances in preventing the disease. For example, some exciting data is emerging from research studies showing that the drug Tamoxifen which is used to treat breast cancer may also play an important role in preventing breast cancer in women deemed to be at high risk to the disease (Powles *et al.* 1990).

Meanwhile there is much to be done to help relieve the psychological distress and dysfunction produced by the diagnosis and treatment. The experiences of women unfortunate enough to have breast cancer which have formed the substance of this book, show that there is little room for complacency. Many women display quite extraordinary fortitude and courage during the course of their disease; others find that the disease exposes the limitations of their coping repertoires. We could all do very much more to make their burden more tolerable.

References

Chapter one

Adjuvant Chemotherapy for Breast Cancer (1985) National Institutes of Health Consensus Development Conference Statements 5 (12).

Berstock, D. A., Houghton, J., Haybittle, J. and Baum, M. (1985) 'The role of radiotherapy following total mastectomy for patients with early breast cancer', *World J Surg* 9:667–70.

Cancer Research Campaign Factsheets (1988).

Fallowfield, L. J., Hall, A., Maguire, G. P. and Baum, M. (1990) 'Psychological outcomes of different treatment policies in women with early breast cancer outside a clinical trial', *BMJ* 301:575–80.

Fisher, B., Bauer, M., Margolese, R. *et al.* (1985) 'Five year results of a randomised clinical trial comparing total mastectomy and segmental mastectomy with or without radiation in the treatment of breast cancer', *N Eng J Med* 312 (11):665–73.

Locker, A. P., Ellis, I. O., Morgan, D. *et al.* (1989) 'Factors influencing local recurrence after excision and radiotherapy for primary breast cancer', *Br J Surg* 76:890–4.

Stoll, B. A. (ed.) (1980) *Women at High Risk to Breast Cancer*, Dordrecht: Kluwer Academic Publishers.

Chapter two

American Cancer Society (1973) *Women's Attitudes Regarding Breast Cancer*, Princeton: The Gallup Organisation.

Briggs, J. E. and Wakefield, J. (1966) *Public Opinion on Cancer: A Survey of Knowledge and Attitudes among Women in Lancaster*, Manchester: Manchester Regional Committee on Cancer.

Calnan, M. (1984) 'The health belief model and participation in programmes for the early detection of cancer: a comparative analysis', *Soc Sci Med* 19 (8):823–30.

References

Calnan, M. (1985) 'Patterns in preventive behaviour: a study of women in middle age', *Soc Sci Med* 20 (3):263–8.

Calnan, M., Chamberlain, J. and Moss, S. (1983) 'Compliance with a class teaching breast self-examination: the impact of the class on the practice of BSE and on women's beliefs about breast cancer', *J Epidemiol Communit Hlth* 37:264–70.

Chamberlain, J., Rogers, P., Price, J. L. *et al.* (1975) 'Validity of clinical examination and mammography as screening tests for breast cancer', *Lancet* (ii):1026–30.

Chilvers, C., McPherson, K., Peto, J., Pike, M. N. and Vessey, M. P. for the UK National Case-Control Study Group (1989) 'Oral contraceptive use and breast cancer risk in young women', *Lancet* (i):973–80.

Cooper, C. L., Cooper, R. and Faragher, B. (1989) 'Incidence and perception of psychosocial stress: the relationship with breast cancer', *Psychol Med* 19:415–22.

Department of Health and Social Security (1986) 'Breast cancer screening', *London HMSO* (Forrest Report).

Duffy, J. C. and Owens, R. G. (1984) 'Factors affecting promptness of reporting in breast cancer patients', *Hygie: International J Health Ed* 3: 29–32.

Ewertz, M. (1986) 'Bereavement and breast cancer', *Br J Ca* 53:701–3.

Fallowfield, L. J., Hall, A., Maguire, G. P. and Baum, M. (1990) 'Psychological outcomes of different treatment policies in women with early breast cancer outside a clinical trial', *BMJ* 301:575–80.

Fallowfield, L. J., Rodway, A. and Baum, M. (1990) 'What are the psychological factors influencing attendance, non-attendance, and reattendance at a breast cancer screening centre?' *JRSM* 83:547–51.

Fink, R., Shapiro, S. and Lewison, J. (1968) 'The reluctant participant in a breast cancer screening programme', *Public Health Rep* 83:479–90.

Fishbein, M. and Ajzen, I. (1975) *Belief, Attitude, Intention and Behaviour. An Introduction to Theory and Research*, Boston: Addison-Western.

Foster, R. S. and Costanza, M. C. (1984) 'Breast self-examination practices and breast cancer survival', *Ca* 53:167–73.

French, K., Porter, A. M. D., Robinson, S. E. *et al* (1982) 'Attendance at a breast screening clinic: a problem of administration or attitudes', *BMJ* 285:617–20.

Gold, M. A. (1964) 'Causes of patients' delay in diseases of the breast', *Ca* 17:564–77.

Grossarth-Maticek, R., Eysenck, H. J., Vetter, H. and Schmidt, P. (1989) 'Psychosocial types and chronic diseases: results of the Heidelberg Prospective Psychosomatic Intervention Study', in S. Maes, C. D. Spielberger, P. B. Defares and I. G. Sarason (eds) *Topics in Health Psychology*, Chichester: John Wiley & Sons Ltd.

Haran, D., Hobbs, P. and Pendleton, L. L. (1979) 'An evaluation of a programme teaching breast self-examination for the early detection of breast cancer', in D. J. Osborne, M. M. Gruneberg and J. R. Eiser (eds) *Research in Psychology and Medicine*, London: Academic Press.

Hobbs, P., Eardley, A. and Wakefield, J. (1977) 'Motivation and education in breast cancer screening', *Pub Health* 91:249–52.

Hobbs, P., George, W. D. and Sellwood, R. A. (1980) 'Characteristics of acceptors and rejectors of breast screening for cancer', *J Epid & Comm Health* 34:19–22.

Hobbs, P., Haran, D. W. and Pendleton, L. L. (1981) 'Breast screening by breast self-examination: an evaluation of teaching methods and materials', *Cancer Detect Prevent* 4:545–51.

Hu, D. and Silberfarb, P. M. (1988) 'Psychological factors: do they influence breast cancer?', in C. L. Cooper (ed.) *Stress and Breast Cancer*, Chichester: John Wiley & Sons Ltd.

Hunt, S. M., Alexander, F. and Maureen Roberts, M. (1988) 'Attenders and non-attenders at a breast screening clinic: a comparative study', *Public Health* 102:3–10.

Knopf, A. (1974) *Cancer: Changes in Opinion after 7 years of Public Education in Lancaster*, Manchester: Manchester Regional Committee on Cancer.

Kroode, H., Oosterwijk, M. and Steverink, N. (1989) 'Three conflicts as a result of causal attributions', *Soc Sci Med* 28:93–7.

McEwen, J., King, E. and Bickler, G. (1989) 'Attendance and non-attendance at the South East London Breast Screening Service', *BMJ* 299:104–6.

MacLean, V., Sinfield, D., Klein, S. and Harnden, B. (1984) 'Women who decline breast screening', *J Epid & Comm Health* 38:278–83.

Mant, D., Vessey, M. P., Neil, A., McPherson, K. and Jones, L. (1987) 'Breast self-examination and breast cancer stage at diagnosis', *Br J Ca* 55:207–11.

Maureen Roberts, M. (1989) 'Breast screening: time for a rethink?', *BMJ* 299:1153–5.

Morris, T. and Greer, S. (1982) 'Psychological characteristics of women electing to attend a breast screening clinic', *J Clin Oncol* 8:113–19.

Owens, R. G., Daly, J. and Heron, K. (1987) 'Psychological and social characteristics of attenders for breast screening', *Psychol & Health* 1:303–13.

Paget, J. (1870) *Surgical Pathology*, London: Longmans Green.

Peters, L. J. and Mason, K. A. (1979) 'Influence of stress on experimental cancer', in B. A. Stoll (ed.) *Mind and Cancer Prognosis*, New York: John Wiley & Sons Ltd.

Peters-Golden, H. (1982) 'Breast cancer: varied perceptions of social support in the illness experience', *Soc Sci Med* 16:483–91.

Priestman, T. J., Priestman, S. G. and Bradshaw, C. (1985) 'Stress and breast cancer', *Br J Ca* 51:493–8.

Rosenstock, I. (1974) 'The health belief model and preventative health behaviour', *Health Educ Mono* 2:354.

Rutledge, D. N., Hartmann, W. H. and Kinman, P. O. (1988) 'Exploration of factors affecting mammography behaviours', *Prevent Med* 17: 412–22.

Sattin, R. W., Rubin, G. L., Webster, L. A. *et al.* (1985) 'Family history and the risk of breast cancer', *JAMA* 253:1908–13.

References

Schonfield, J. (1975) 'Psychological and life-experience differences between Israeli women with benign and cancerous breast lesions', *J Psychosom Res* 19:229–34.

Smith, E. M., Francis, A. M. and Polissar, L. (1980) 'The effect of breast self-examination practices and physician examinations on extent of disease at diagnosis', *Prevent Med* 9:409–17.

Snow, H. L. (1893) *Cancer and the Cancer Process*, London: Churchill.

Stillman, M. J. (1977) 'Women's health beliefs about breast cancer and breast self-examination', *Nurs Res* 26 (2):121–7.

Turnbull, E. M. (1978) 'Effect of basic preventive health practices and mass media on the practice of breast self-examination', *Nurs Res* 27:98–102.

Verres, R. (1986) *Krebs und Angst. Subjektive Theorien uber Ursachen, Verhutung, Fruherkennung, Behandlung und die psychosozialen Folgen von Krebserkrankungen*, Berlin, Heidelberg: Springer-Verlag.

Chapter three

Aiken-Swan, J. and Paterson, R. (1955) 'The cancer patient: delay in seeking medical advice', *BMJ* (i):623–7.

Buttlar, C. H. and Templeton, A. C. (1983) 'The size of breast masses at presentation: the impact of prior medical training', *Ca* 51:1750–3.

Cameron, A. and Hinton, J. (1968) 'Delay in seeking treatment for mammary tumours', *Ca* 21:1121–6.

Cassileth, B. R., Lusk, E. J., Strousse, T. B. *et al.* (1985) 'A psychological analysis of cancer patients and their next of kin', *Ca* 55:72–6.

Eardley, A. and Wakefield, J. (1976) 'Lay consultation by women with a lump in the breast', *Br Med J* 2:33–9.

Ellman, R. (1989) 'Clinical cost-benefit of screening programmes', in B. A. Stoll (ed.) *Women at High Risk to Breast Cancer*, Dordrecht: Kluwer Academic Publishers.

Fallowfield, L. J., Baum, M. and Maguire, G. P. (1987) 'Addressing the psychological needs of the conservatively treated breast cancer patient: discussion paper', *JRSM* 80:696–700.

Fallowfield, L. J., Hall, A., Maguire, G. P. and Baum, M. (1990) 'Psychological outcomes of different treatment policies in women with early breast cancer outside a clinical trial', *BMJ* 301:575–80.

Frankel, M. R. (1988) 'Breast cancer – a woman's perspective', *West J Med* 149:723–5.

Frankel, M. R. and Canepa, L. (1988) 'Telling your kids you have cancer or any serious illness', *Med Self-Care*, September-October:37–41.

Gates, C. C. (1980) 'Husbands of mastectomy patients', *Patient Counselling & Health Educ* 1:38–41.

Gold, M. A. (1964) 'Causes of patients' delay in diseases of the breast', *Ca* 17:564–77.

Greer, S. (1974) 'Psychological aspects: delay in the treatment of breast cancer', *Proceedings of the RSM* 67:470–3.

Hogbin, B. and Fallowfield, L. J. (1989) 'Getting it taped: the "bad news" consultation with cancer patients', *Br J Hosp Med* 41:330–3.

Hughes, J. (1987) *Cancer and Emotion. Psychological Preludes and Reactions to Cancer*, Chichester: John Wiley & Sons Ltd.

Knopf, A. (1974) *Cancer: Changes in Opinion after 7 years of Public Education in Lancaster*, Manchester: Manchester Regional Committee on Cancer.

Lewis, F. M., Ellison, E. S. and Woods, N. F. (1985) 'The impact of breast cancer on the family', *Semin Oncol Nurs* 3:206–13.

Ley, P. and Spelman, M. S. (1965) 'Communications in an out-patient setting', *Br J Soc & Clin Psychol* 4:114–16.

Ley, P. and Spelman, M. S. (1967) *Communicating with the Patient*, London: Saples Press.

Lichtman, R. R., Taylor, S. E., Wood, J. F. *et al.* (1984) 'Relations with children after breast cancer: the mother-daughter relationship at risk', *J Psychosoc Oncol* 2 (3/4):1–19.

Maguire, G. P. (1976) 'The psychological and social sequelae of mastectomy', in J. Howell (ed.) *Modern Perspectives in the Psychiatric Aspects of Surgery*, New York: Brunei Mayel: 390–421.

Maguire, G. P. (1984) 'Can the parental psychological morbidity associated with childhood leukaemia be reduced?', *Cancer Surveys* 3:617–31.

Margarey, C. J., Todd, P. B. and Blizzard, P. J. (1977) 'Psychosocial factors influencing delay and breast self-examination in women with symptoms of breast cancer', *Soc Sci Med* 11:229–32.

Morris, T., Greer, H. S. and White, P. (1977) 'Psychological and social adjustment to mastectomy', *Ca* 40:2381–7.

Morton, J. (1987) 'Personal view', *BMJ* 295:1482.

Plumb, M. and Holland, J. (1977) 'Comparative studies of psychological function in patients with advanced cancer – Self-reported depressive symptoms', *Psychosom Med* 39 (4):264–76.

Ray, C. and Baum, M. (1985) *Psychological Aspects of Early Breast Cancer*, New York: Springer-Verlag.

Renneker, R. and Cutler, M. (1952) 'Psychological problems of adjustment to cancer of the breast', *JAMA* 148:833–8.

Sabo, D., Brown, J. and Smith, C. (1986) 'The male role and mastectomy: support groups and men's adjustment', *J Psychosoc Oncol* 4:19–31.

Scott, D. W. (1983) 'Anxiety, critical thinking and information processing during and after breast biopsy', *Nurs Res* 32:24–9.

Wellisch, D. K. (1979) 'Adolescent acting out when a parent has cancer', *Int Fam Ther* 1:230–41.

Williams, E. M., Baum, M. and Hughes, L. E. (1976) 'Delay in presentation of women with breast disease', *Clin Oncol* 2:327–31.

Chapter four

Ashcroft, J. J., Leinster, S. J. and Slade, P. D. (1985) 'Breast cancer – patient choice of treatment: preliminary communication', *J Roy Soc Med* 78:43–6.

References

Bard, M. and Sutherland, A. M. (1955) 'Psychological impact of cancer and its treatment IV: adaptation to radical mastectomy', *Ca* 8:652–72.

Baric, L. (1969) 'Recognition of the "at risk" role: a means to influence health behaviour', *Int J Health Ed* 12:24–34.

Bartelink, H., van Dam, F. and van Dongen, J. (1985) 'Psychological effects of breast conserving therapy in comparison with radical mastectomy', *Int J Radiation Oncol Biol Phys* 11:381–5.

Dean, C. (1987) 'Psychiatric morbidity following mastectomy', *J Psychosom Res* 31:385–92.

Dean, C., Chetty, V. and Forrest, A. P. M. (1983) 'Effects of immediate breast reconstruction on psychosocial morbidity after mastectomy', *Lancet* i:459–62.

Fallowfield, L. J., Baum, M. and Maguire, G. P. (1986) 'Effects of breast conservation on psychological morbidity associated with diagnosis and treatment of early breast cancer', *BMJ* 293:1331–4.

Fallowfield, L. J., Baum, M. and Maguire, G. P. (1987) 'Addressing the psychological needs of the conservatively treated breast cancer patient: discussion paper', *JRSM* 80:696–700.

Fallowfield, L. J., Hall, A., Maguire, G. P. and Baum, M. (1990) 'Psychological outcomes of different treatment policies in women with early breast cancer outside a clinical trial', *BMJ* 301:575–80.

Fisher, B., Bauer, M., Margolese, R. *et al.* (1985) 'Five year results of a randomised clinical trial comparing total mastectomy and segmental mastectomy with or without radiation in the treatment of breast cancer', *N Eng J Med* 312 (11):665–73.

de Haes, J. C. J. M., van Oostrom, M. A. and Welvaart, K. (1986) 'The effect of radical and conserving surgery on the quality of life of early breast cancer patients', *Eur J Surg Oncol* 12:337–42.

Hall, A. and Fallowfield, L. J. (1989) 'Psychological outcome of treatment for early breast cancer: a review', *Stress Med* 5:167–75.

Jamison, K. R., Wellisch, D. K. and Pasnau, R. O. (1978) 'Psychosocial aspects of mastectomy I: the woman's perspective', *Amer J Psych* 135:432–6.

Kemeny, M. M., Wellisch, D. K. and Schain, W. S. (1988) 'Psychosocial outcome in a randomised surgical trial for treatment of primary breast cancer', *Ca* 62:1231–7.

Lasry, J. C. M., Margolese, R. G., Poisson, R. *et al.* (1987) 'Depression and body image following mastectomy and lumpectomy', *J Chron Dis* 40 (6): 529–34.

Lucas, D., Maguire, G. P., Reason, J. *et al.* (1987) 'Predicting psychiatric morbidity in women with breast cancer', *Report to the North West Region Health Authority*, Manchester.

Maguire, G. P. (1985) 'The psychological and social consequences of breast cancer', *Nurs Mirror* 140:540–7.

Maguire, G. P. (1989) 'Breast conservation versus mastectomy: psychological considerations', *Sem in Surg Oncol* 5:137–44.

Maguire, G. P., Lee, E. G., Bevington, D. J. *et al.* (1978) 'Psychiatric problems in the first year after mastectomy', *BMJ* (i):963–5.

126

Maguire, G. P., Tait, A., Brooke, M. *et al.* (1980) 'Psychiatric morbidity and physical toxicity associated with adjuvant chemotherapy after mastectomy', *BMJ* (ii):1179–80.

Maunsell, E., Brisson, J. and Deschenes, L. (1989) 'Psychological distress after initial treatment for breast cancer: a comparison of partial and total mastectomy', *J Clin Epidemiol* 42 (8):765–71.

Meyer, L. and Aspergren, K. (1989) 'Long term psychological sequelae of mastectomy and breast conserving treatment for breast cancer', *Acta Oncol* 28:13–18.

Morris, T., Greer, H. S. and White, P. (1977) 'Psychological and social adjustment to mastectomy', *Ca* 40:2381–7.

Morris, J. and Royle, G. J. (1988) 'Offering patients a choice of surgery for early breast cancer: a reduction in anxiety and depression in patients and their husbands', *Soc Sci Med* 26 (6):583–5.

Nolvadex Adjuvant Trial Organisation (1985) 'Controlled trial of tamoxifen as single adjuvant agent in management of early breast cancer. Analysis at six years', *Lancet* (i):836–40.

Parsons, J. A., Webster, J. H. and Dowd, J. E. (1961) 'Evaluation of the placebo effect in the treatment of radiation sickness', *Acta Radiologica* 56:129–40.

Penman, D. T., Bloom, J. R., Fotopolous, S. *et al.* (1987) 'The impact of mastectomy on self-concept and social function: a combined cross-sectional and longitudinal study with comparison groups', in S. Stellman (ed.) *Women and Cancer*, New York: The Haworth Press Inc.

Prior, A. (1988) 'How I kept my breast despite cancer', *Independent Newspaper*, 2 February.

Ray, C. and Baum, M. (1985) *Psychological Aspects of Early Breast Cancer*, New York: Springer-Verlag.

Renneker, R. and Cutler, M. (1952) 'Psychological problems of adjustment to cancer of the breast', *JAMA* 148:833–8.

Sanger, C. K. and Reznikoff, M. (1981) 'A comparison of the psychological effects of breast-saving procedures with the modified radical mastectomy', *Ca* 48:2341–6.

Schain, W., Edwards, B. K., Gorrell, C. R. *et al.* (1983) 'Psychosocial and physical outcomes of primary breast cancer therapy: mastectomy vs. excisional biopsy and irradiation', *Br Ca Res Treat* 3:377–82.

Schover, L. R. and Jensen, S.B. (1988) *Sexuality and Chronic Illness. A Comprehensive Approach*, New York: The Guildford Press.

Silberfarb, P. M., Maurer, H. L. and Crouthamel, C. S. (1980) 'Psychosocial aspects of neoplastic disease I: functional status of breast cancer patients during different treatment regimens', *Am J Psych* 137 (4):450–5.

Silberfarb, P. M., Philibert, D. and Levine, P. M. (1980) 'Psychosocial aspects of neoplastic disease II: affective and cognitive effects of chemotherapy in cancer patients', *Am J Psych* 137 (5):597–601.

Steinberg, M. D., Juliano, M. S. and Wise, L. (1985) 'Psychological outcome of lumpectomy versus mastectomy in the treatment of breast cancer', *Am J Psychiat* 142:34–9.

Tarrier, N. (1987) *Living with Breast Cancer and Mastectomy*, Manchester: Manchester University Press.

Valanis, B. G. and Rumpler, C. H. (1985) 'Helping women to choose breast cancer treatment alternatives', *Cancer Nurs* 8:167–75.

Veronesi, U., Saccozzi, R., Del Veahio, M. *et al* (1981) 'Comparing radical mastectomy with quadrantectomy, axillary dissection and radiotherapy in patients with small cancers of the breast', *N Eng J Med* 305 (1):6–11.

Wabrek, A. J. and Wabrek, C. J. (1976) 'Mastectomy: sexual implications', *Primary Care* 3:803.

Wolberg, W. H., Tanner, M. A., Romsaas, E. P. *et al* (1987) 'Factors influencing options in primary breast cancer treatment', *J Clin Oncol* 5 (1) Jan: 68–74.

Chapter five

American Cancer Society (1983) 'Unproven methods of cancer management', *Macrobiotic Diets*, New York: ACS.

Baum, M. (1986) 'Alternative medicine and oncology in the United Kingdom', *Cancer Topics* 5:135–6.

Baum, M. (1989) 'Rationalism versus irrationalism in the care of the sick: science versus the absurd', *Med J Aust* 151:607–8.

Bukberg, J., Penman, D. and Holland, J. C. (1984) 'Depression in hospitalised cancer patients', *Psychosom Med* 46:199–212.

Cassileth, B. R. (1986) 'Unorthodox cancer medicine', *Cancer Invest* 4 (6): 591–8.

Clark, A. and Fallowfield, L. J. (1986) 'Quality of life measurements in patients with malignant disease', *J Roy Soc Med* 79:165–9.

Fallowfield, L. J. and Baum, M. (1989) 'Psychological welfare of patients with breast cancer', *J Roy Soc Med* 82:4–5.

Fallowfield, L. J. (1990) *The Quality of Life: the Missing Measurement in Health Care*, London: Souvenir Press.

Goldie, L. (1982) 'The ethics of telling the patient', *J Med Ethics* 8:128–33.

Gotay, C. C. (1984) 'The experience of cancer during early and advanced stages: the views of patients and their mates', *Soc Sci Med* 18: 605–13.

Holland, J. C. (1977) 'Psychological aspects of oncology', *Med Clin of N America* 61:737–48.

Holland, J. C. and Rowland, J. H. (1989) *Handbook of Psycho-oncology. Psychological Care of the Patient with Cancer*, New York: Oxford University Press, 513.

Hopwood, P. (1984) 'Measurement of psychological morbidity in cancer', in M. Watson and S. Greer (eds) *Psychosocial Issues in Malignant Disease*, Oxford: Pergamon Press.

Lerner, M. (1985) 'A report on complementary cancer therapies. Advances', *J Inst Advanc Health* 2 (1):31–43.

Lloyd, G. (1979) 'Psychological stress and coping: mechanisms in patients with cancer', in B. A. Stoll (ed.) *Mind and Cancer Prognosis*, New York: John Wiley & Sons Ltd.

Massie, M. J., Holland, J. C. and Glass, E. (1983) 'Delirium in terminally ill cancer patients', *Am J Psychiat* 140:1048–50.

Plumb, M. and Holland, J. (1977) 'Comparative studies of psychological function in patients with advanced cancer – self-reported depressive symptoms', *Psychosom Med* 39:264–76.

Plumb, M. and Holland, J. (1981) 'Comparative studies of psychological function in patients with advanced cancer II: interviewer rated current and past psychiatric symptoms', *Psychosom Med* 43:243–54.

Ramirez, A. J., Craig, T. K. J., Watson, J. P. *et al.* (1989) 'Stress and relapse of breast cancer', *Br Med J* 298:291–3.

Redding, K. L., Beutler, S., Jones, F. *et al.* (1981) 'Psychosocial attitudes of cancer patients treated with laetrile or other phase II agents', *Proc 72nd Ann Mtg Am Assoc Ca Res C-243* 22:394.

Rorsch, P. (1981) 'Stress: cause or cure of cancer?', in J. Goldberg (ed.) *Psychotherapeutic treatment of cancer patients*, New York: Free Press.

Silberfarb, P. M., Maurer, H. L. and Grouthamel, C. S. (1980) 'Psychosocial aspects of neoplastic disease I: Functional status of breast cancer patients during different treatment regimens', *Am J Psych* 137: (4):450–5.

Simonton, O. C., Simonton, S. and Creighton, J. L. (1980) *Getting Well Again*, New York: Bantam Books.

Welsman, A. D. and Worden, J. W. (1986) 'The emotional impact of recurrent cancer', *J Psychosoc Oncol* 3:5–16.

Chapter six

Anderson, C. R. (1977) 'Locus of control, coping behaviours and performance in a stress setting: a longitudinal study', *J Appl Psychiatry* 62:446–51.

Bard, J. R. (1982) 'Social support, accommodation to stress and adjustment to breast cancer', *Soc Sci Med* 16:1329–38.

Bard, M. and Sutherland, A. M. (1955) 'Psychological impact of cancer and its treatment', *Ca* 8:656–72.

Bloom, J. R. (1982) 'Social support, accommodation to stress and adjustment to breast cancer', *Soc Sci Med* 16:1329–38.

Burish, T. G. and Lyles, J. N. (1981) 'Effectiveness of relaxation training in reducing adverse reactions to cancer chemotherapy', *J Behavioural Med* 4:65–78.

Cella, D. F., Pratt, A. and Holland, J. C. (1986) 'Persistent anticipatory nausea, vomiting and anxiety in cured Hodgkin's disease patients after completion of chemotherapy', *Am J Psychiatry* 143:641–3.

Cunningham, A. (1988) 'From neglect to support to coping. The evolution of psychosocial intervention for cancer patients', in C. L. Cooper (ed.) *Stress and Breast Cancer*, Chichester: John Wiley & Sons Ltd.

Dunkel-Schetter, C. (1984) 'Social support and cancer: findings based on patient interviews and their implications', *J Soc Issues* 40:77–9.

Ell, K. O., Mantell, J. E. and Hamaritch, M. B. (1989) 'Social support, sense of control and coping among patients with breast, lung or colorectal cancer', *J Psychosoc Oncol* 7 (3):63–89.

Fallowfield, L. J. (1988) 'Counselling for patients with cancer', *BMJ* 297:727–8.

Fallowfield, L. J., Baum, M. and Maguire, G. P. (1987) 'Addressing the psychological needs of the conservatively treated breast cancer patient: discussion paper', *JRSM* 80:696–700.

Fallowfield, L. J., Baum, M. and Maguire, G. P. (1987) 'Do psychological studies upset patients', *JRSM* 80:59.

Fallowfield, L. J. and Roberts, R. (1992) 'Cancer counselling in the United Kingdom', *Psychology & Health* 6:107–17.

Feifel, H., Strack, S. and Nagy, V. T. (1987) 'Coping strategies and associated features of medically ill patients', *Psychosom Med* 49:616–25.

Funch, D. P. and Mettlin, C. (1982) 'The role of support in relation to recovery from breast surgery', *Soc Sci Med* 16:91–8.

Greer, S., Morris, T. and Pettingale, K. W. (1979) 'Psychological response to breast cancer: effect on outcome', *Lancet* (ii):785–7.

Holland, J. C., Rowland, J., Lebovits, A. and Rusalem, R. (1979) 'Reactions to cancer treatment: assessment of emotional response to adjuvant radiotherapy as a guide to planned intervention', *Psychiatric Clin of N Am* 2 (2):347–58.

Jamison, K. R., Wellisch, D. K. and Pasnau, R. O. (1978) 'Psychosocial aspects of mastectomy I: the woman's perspective', *Am J Psych* 135:432–6.

Knobf, T. (1986) 'Physical and psychologic distress associated with adjuvant chemotherapy in women with breast cancer', *J Clin Oncol* 4:678–84.

Lazarus, R. S. and Folkman, S. (1984) *Stress Appraisal and Coping*, New York: Springer.

Lerner, M. J. and Miller, D. T. (1978) 'Just world research and the attribution process: looking back and ahead', *Psychol Bull* 85:1030–51.

Lipowski, Z. J. (1970) 'Physical illness, the individual and the coping processes', *Psychiatry Med* 1:91–102.

Maguire, G. P., Tait, A., Brooks, M., Thomas, C. and Sellwood, R. (1980) 'Effect of counselling on the psychiatric morbidity associated with mastectomy', *BMJ* (ii):1454–6.

Mantell, J. E. (1983) 'Cancer patient visitor programs: a case for accountability, *J Psychosoc Oncol* 1:45–58.

Mastrovito, R., Moynihan, R. and Parsonnet, L. (1989) 'Self-help and mutual support programs', in J. C. Holland and J. Rowland (eds) *Handbook of Psycho-oncology*, New York: Oxford University Press: 502–7.

Meyerowitz, V. W., Watkins, I. K. and Sparks, F. C. (1983) 'Psychosocial implications of adjuvant chemotherapy. A two-year follow-up', *Ca* 52:1541–5.

Moss, R. H. and Schaefer, J. A. (1984) 'The crisis of physical illness. An overview and conceptual approach', in R. H. Moss (ed.) *Coping with Physical Illness* vol. 2:3–25.

Nichols, K. (1989) Personal communication.

Penman, D. T. (1982) 'Coping strategies in adaptation to mastectomy', *Psychosom Med* 44:117.

Penman, D. T., Holland, J. C., Bahna, G. *et al.* (1984) 'Informed consent for investigational chemotherapy. Patients' and physicians' perceptions', *J Clin Oncol* 2:849–55.

Peters-Golden, H. (1982) 'Breast cancer: varied perceptions of social support in the illness experience', *Soc Sci Med* 16:483–91.

Plant, H., Richardson, J., Stubbs, L. *et al.* (1987) 'Evaluation of a support group for cancer patients and their families and friends', *Br J Hosp Med* 38 (4):317–22.

Redd, W. H., Anderson, G. V. and Minagawa, R. Y. (1982) 'Hypnotic control of anticipatory emesis in patients receiving cancer chemotherapy', *J Consulting & Clin Psychol* 50:14–19.

Reissman, F. (1965) 'The 'helper-therapy' principle', *Soc Work* 10:27–32.

Roberts, R. and Fallowfield, L. J. (1990) 'Who supports the cancer counsellors?', *Nurs. Times* 86(36):32–4.

Spiegel, D., Bloom, J., Kraemer, H. and Gottheil, E. (1989) 'Effect of psychosocial treatment on survival of patients with metastatic breast cancer', *Lancet*, October:888–90.

Van Komen, R. and Redd, W. H. (1985) 'Personality factors associated with anticipatory nausea/vomiting in patients receiving cancer chemotherapy', *Health Psychol* 4:189–202.

Watson, M. (1983) 'Psychosocial intervention with cancer patients: a review', *Psychol Med* 13:839–46.

Watson, M., Denton, S., Baum, M. and Greer, S. (1988) 'Counselling breast cancer patients: a specialist nurse service', *Counselling Psychol Quarterly* 1 (1):25–34.

Chapter seven

Ashcroft, J. J., Leinster, S. J. and Slade, P. D. (1985) 'Breast cancer: patient choice of treatment', *JRSM* 78:43.

Cassileth, B. R., Zupkiss, R. V., Sutton-Smith, K. and March, V. (1980) 'Information and participation preferences among cancer patients', *Annals Int Med* 92:832–6.

Clements, C. D. and Sider, R. C. (1983) 'Medical ethics' assault upon medical values', *J Am Med Assoc* 205:2011–15.

Fallowfield, L. J., Hall, A., Maguire, G. P. and Baum, M. (1990) 'Psychological outcomes of different treatment policies in women with early breast cancer outside a clinical trial', *BMJ* 301:575–80.

Hershey, J. C. and Baron, J. (1987) 'Clinical reasoning and cognitive processes', *Med Decis Making* 7:203–11.

Katz, J. (1984) *The Silent World of Doctor and Patient*, New York: The Free Press.

Locker, A. P., Ellis, I. O., Morgan, D. A. L. *et al.* (1989) 'Factors influencing local recurrence after excision and radiotherapy for primary breast cancer', *Br J Surg* 76:890–4.

Morris, J., Royle, G. T. and Taylor, I. (1989) 'Changes in the surgical management of early breast cancer in England', *JRSM* 82 (1):12–14.

Powles, T.J., Tillyer, C.R., Jones, A.L. *et al.* (1990) 'Prevention of breast cancer with Tamoxifen – an update on the Royal Marsden Hospital pilot programme', *Eur J Ca* 26 (6):680–4.

Schoene-Seifert, B. and Childress, J. R. (1986) 'How much should the cancer patient know and decide', *Ca-A Ca J for Clinicians* 36:85–94.

Sutherland, H. J., Llewellyn-Thomas, H. A., Lockwood, G. A., Tritchler, D. L. and Till, J. E. (1989) 'Cancer patients: their desire for information and participation in treatment decisions', *J Roy Soc Med* 82 (5):260–3.

Wagener, J. J. and Taylor, S. E. (1986) 'What else could I have done? Patients' responses to failed treatment decisions', *Health Psychol* 5 (5): 481–96.

Index